What Celebrities Are Saying About Scott-Vincent Borba

"Scott-Vincent Borba's philosophy about treating your inner health as much as your outer health is paramount to healthy living."

—**Paula Abdul**, *American Idol* and *Got to Dance*

"I love Scott-Vincent Borba!"

—**Nancy O'Dell**, *Access Hollywood, Today Show, Dateline NBC,* and *Your OWN Show: Oprah's Search for the Next TV Star*

"His methods work better than most because he thinks outside of the box. It's not the standard creams and lotions and cleansing. Everything is about beauty from the inside out. He is awesome and knows everything there is to know about skin care."

—**Jayde Nicole**, *The Hills*

"Scott-Vincent Borba is so inspirational, and I was very impressed with him . . . and the fact that he comes from a science-based background is fantastic."

—**Mila Kunis**, *That '70s Show, Family Guy,* and *Forgetting Sarah Marshall*

"He's a genius!"

—**Lucy Hale**, *Pretty Little Liars* and *Privileged*

"He has such incredibly amazing skin, and what he's doing for skin care is wonderful!"

—**Lynn Collins**, *X-Men Origins: Wolverine,* and *The Merchant of Venice*

"I've learned so much from Scott-Vincent Borba. His inside-out philosophy about skin care is something I absolutely connect to and really believe in. He's amazing."

—**Stacy Keibler**, actress

"Scott-Vincent's work, products, lifestyle, and overall glow reaffirmed my belief that eating well and living with joy manifests itself on your outer being. BORBA is really an amazing skin-care line. The purity of the product and the innovative techniques make Scott-Vincent my new hero! After using BORBA, you won't believe your face—it will simply amaze you!"

—**Brittany Ishibashi**, *The Bannen Way*
and *Ghostfacers* web series

"When it comes to skin care, Scott-Vincent is more knowledgeable than many dermatologists! It's nice that I can go to someone who's really studying the human body and noticing the effects that certain things have, as far as what you're taking in and what you're putting on topically."

—**AnnaLynne McCord**, *90210* and *Nip/Tuck*

skintervention™

The Personalized Solution for Healthier, Younger, and Flawless-Looking Skin

Scott-Vincent Borba™
with **Debbie Appel**

Health Communications, Inc.
Deerfield Beach, Florida

www.hcibooks.com

The information contained in this publication is not intended to replace the services of a physician, nor does it constitute a doctor-patient relationship. All content in this publication is provided for informational purposes, and readers should consult their own physicians concerning any recommendations.

You should not use the information in this publication for diagnosing or treating a medical or health condition. If you have or suspect you have an urgent medical problem, promptly contact your professional healthcare provider. Any application of the suggestions in this publication is at the reader's discretion.

Library of Congress Cataloging-in-Publication Data

Borba, Scott-Vincent.
    Skintervention : the personalized solution for healthier, younger, and flawless-looking skin / Scott-Vincent Borba.
      p. cm.
    Includes index.
    ISBN-13: 978-0-7573-1552-7
    ISBN-10: 0-7573-1552-6
    1. Skin—Care and hygiene. 2. Beauty, Personal. I. Title. II. Title: Skin intervention.

RL87.B662 2011
646.7'26—dc22

2010039145

Publisher: Health Communications, Inc.
    3201 S.W. 15th Street
    Deerfield Beach, FL 33442–8190

Cover design by Justin Rotkowitz
Interior design and formatting by Lawna Patterson Oldfield

Celebrities Love Scott-Vincent Borba!

In addition to Scott-Vincent Borba's line of mass-market nutraceutical and cosmeceutical products, he has also developed an amazing reputation as a skin-care expert in the entertainment world, resulting from the success his many celebrity clients have achieved. Some of his glowing clients include:

★ Mila Kunis of *That '70s Show*, *Family Guy*, and *Forgetting Sarah Marshall*

★ Ashley Greene of *Twilight*, *Twilight: New Moon*, and *Twilight: Eclipse*

★ Nancy O'Dell of *Access Hollywood*, *Today Show*, and *Dateline NBC*

★ Lucy Hale of *Pretty Little Liars* and *Privileged*

★ AnnaLynne McCord of *90210* and *Nip/Tuck*

★ Ed Quinn of *Eureka* and *True Blood*

★ Jayde Nicole of *The Hills*

★ Brooke Nevin of *Imaginary Bitches* and *The 4400*

★ Lynn Collins of *X-Men Origins: Wolverine* and *The Merchant of Venice*

★ Brittany Ishibashi of *The Bannen Way* and *Ghostfacers* web series

★ Kimberly Elise of *Close to Home* and *Diary of a Mad Black Woman*

★ Arielle Kebbel of *Vampires Suck* and *John Tucker Must Die*

Some of his enthusiastic fans include:

★ Paula Abdul of *American Idol* and *Got to Dance*

★ Billy Bush of *Access Hollywood*

★ Selena Gomez of *Wizards of Waverly Place* and *Ramona and Beezus*

★ Cloris Leachman of *You Again* and *The Women*

★ Haylie Duff of *7th Heaven* and *Material Girls*

★ Jack McBrayer of *30 Rock* and *Forgetting Sarah Marshall*

★ Stacy Keibler, actress

★ Jennifer Carpenter of *Dexter* and *Quarantine*

★ James Kyson-Lee of *Heroes* and *Shutter*

★ Rachelle Lefevre of *Twilight* and *Twilight: New Moon*

★ Maureen McCormick of *The Brady Bunch*

★ Adam Arkin of *Sons of Anarchy* and *Life*

This book is dedicated to
my beloved father and mother who have
supported and nurtured my creative vision from the
start, and to the faith they instilled in me.

I also dedicate this book to Jesus and the Virgin Mary,
as without prayer I would not have the inspiration
to wake up each day to push forward to help change
people's lives in holistic and spiritual ways.

Finally, this book is dedicated to any of
you who have ever been told "no" to your dreams.
You wouldn't be reading this now if I had listened
to all the people who said "no" to me.
I wholeheartedly support you and your vision.
Go after your dreams—you **can** make them a reality.
It all starts now with YOU!

Contents

· ·

Foreword

THE DAY I MET SCOTT-VINCENT BORBA and discovered what he was all about, I knew my life would be changed for the better. His passion, exuberance, and incredible knowledge about skin care made me an instant believer.

I met Scott-Vincent in 2009 when I went to his office for my first treatment. Before that day, I had always stuck to the basics in beauty, since I didn't trust or believe in the complete effectiveness of many of the overmarketed products out there. But Scott-Vincent's philosophy and radically innovative products seemed like the perfect match for what I was searching for in skin care. I told Scott-Vincent that I was hopeful he could help me make my eyes look well rested, keep my skin as porcelain-looking as possible, and show me how to eat the right foods that would reveal my healthiest skin.

After the treatment, I looked and felt absolutely beautiful. The difference in my appearance was incredible. I left his office with a sense of joy because I knew exactly what I needed to do every day, from my diet to the types of ingredients I should look for in my skin-care products. The glow I had on my face that day (and after every time I have had one of his treatments) was so noticeable that I got compliments left and right! And fortunately for me, I am able to maintain that radiance day after day because I follow Scott-Vincent's philosophy and methods for achieving beauty from the inside out.

He is one of the very few, if not the only person who synergizes both the topical and the internal systems to work together. It's an approach that I wholeheartedly believe in and have incorporated into my daily life. I've learned what foods I need to eat to keep my skin beautiful, how to correctly use the right products for my skin type, and what I need to do for proper hydration. And I learned all of this from Scott-Vincent! I also know that if I continue to do those things, I'm going to look and feel the way I need to for my career long-term, and I'll be able to boldly project the confidence I feel internally.

Scott-Vincent Borba's inspired and revitalizing health and skin-care revelations have both enhanced and altered the way I take care of my body and my skin. I am so excited that he's written this book so he can share his vast wealth of skin-care knowledge and brilliant insights with you. So listen to what he has to say, really take his advice to heart, and from firsthand experience, I can promise you that the end results will be well worth it!

—Lucy Hale, actress
ABC Family's *Pretty Little Liars*

Introduction:
Do You Need a **Skin**tervention?

NATURALLY BEAUTIFUL, FLAWLESS SKIN—we all want to
have it, but not everyone knows how to get it, or, more important,
how to maintain it. However, as I learned firsthand, where there's
knowledge, dedication, and action, there's absolutely a way to
make it a reality. I want to share with you everything I discovered
during my eye-opening journey and help you achieve the gorgeous exterior appearance you've been trying so hard to perfect
. . . working from the inside out! Let me start by telling you my
story and how it all began.

When I was a teenager I had terrible cystic acne, a mild case of
rosacea, and I was overweight in all the wrong places. I had no
confidence and felt as if I were the only one in the world with
these problems. Like most people, I wanted to look "roll-out-of-
bed" beautiful and not have to spend hours every day getting
ready, but I had to camouflage things in order to face the world.
When it came to covering up my acne, I became a magician with
Clearasil's tinted acne cream. I figured out how to dab it onto my
skin and rub it in so perfectly that it matched my skin tone

exactly. No one knew by looking at me that I had an array of challenges underneath the surface. But it was exhausting doing that day after day after day!

Ironically, despite my physical insecurities, I fell into a successful career as a product development and marketing specialist in the health and beauty industry. With every new brand or product launch, I changed people's skin for the better, but found myself hiding behind the cameras because I was embarrassed by my horrible complexion. The longer I worked for top luxury skin-care companies dealing with my own challenging skin, the more I realized I had to dig deeper (literally) to find a personal solution.

The catalyst came when my father developed pancreatic cancer. I took a break to care for him and devoted my time to studying the human body, nutraceuticals, and natural ingredients. As I saw how fortifying my father's daily regimen with certain foods and supplements improved his health, energy levels, and the quality of his life, my "aha" moment struck. I realized the same principles could be applied to solving my skin's issues as well. I decided to test my theory. By modifying my diet to include key foods, nutrients, and antioxidants for my skin type, as well as taking some supplements, I saw a dramatic change in my skin for the better.

Then I took it a step further. I discovered that if you combine the foods you ingest internally that target the inner causes of skin complaints with the products you use topically, you enable all of the layers of your skin to work synergistically and soon enough, your skin and cells begin to improve themselves from within. When you nourish your body on the inside *and* outside with foods and products containing the same ingredients, your skin is in perfect communication from your epidermis to the dermal layers, which makes your skin healthier, thereby making it look better. Healthier skin on the inside means healthier skin on the outside! Once I started practicing what I was preaching, the results were undeniable: my skin problems subsided, my confidence returned, and I became an entirely new person!

Energized by my own skin transformation, I began developing products that would fuse topical ingredients with ingestible nutrients—and my line of BORBA products was born. Today, BORBA products are used by some of Hollywood's top celebrities and are available in many well-known retail stores, including Fred Segal, Bloomingdales, CVS Beauty 360, Ulta, and Walgreen's.

By taking my own newfound passion and knowledge and channeling it into helping others, I was able to see the fruits of my labor in the success of those around me. I then turned to other members of my family and some of my closest friends and used them as my first "product testers." They had a variety of skin challenges, and once they implemented this inside-out lifestyle, the changes were incredible. The best part was, it wasn't about forcing them to completely alter their lives, but about how they could make a few tweaks to common things they were already doing in their lives—from the products they used to how they applied them. Given their success, I knew this way of life could work for just about anyone!

Then I obtained my first celebrity client and was under a lot of pressure to eliminate some of her skin issues, which, if not fixed, would be visible to the entire world. I realized that helping her make these internal and external changes would not only help with her career but could also help increase her confidence and maybe get her to the next level . . . and it did! Once she changed a few simple things in her lifestyle, her acne started clearing up, her confidence soared, and she landed a fantastic TV role.

It still gives me goose bumps when I realize that by helping people make the simplest changes in their lives, the way they look and feel about themselves is completely altered . . . the same way it was for me. Now are you ready to start your own journey toward reinventing your skin and the way you see yourself? Staging your own skintervention is as easy as using the food in your pantry properly and making your current skin-care products work for you, not against you.

Your Own Skintervention

So now it's time to focus on you. What do you want? Everyone is different. Maybe you want less wrinkles and younger-looking eyes. Maybe you want clearer skin. You might be confident about your jiggly parts, but you want more radiant skin. Identify what you want to look like and not what society tells you or even what you are projecting onto yourself.

Step back for a second and ask, "When I look in the mirror, what do I want to see? Do I want to see clarity? Do I want to see less aging? Do I want to see myself looking well rested and wide awake? Do I want to look recharged?"

Really decide what *you* want to look like. Whether you want to fix an existing skin problem or just want to look healthier, the key element is to identify what it is—inside and out—and begin your process from there.

To help you make some of those decisions, I'll help you identify a few core issues that may be causing some of your skin challenges: your surroundings, stress levels, food triggers, relationships, and daily habits. Once you recognize how much the everyday things around you affect your skin, you'll be able to readjust and use those things in your daily life.

Even some of the most beautiful Hollywood celebrities are now realizing the power that a few changes can make. One of my A-list clients had challenges with facial acne for years. She recently came to see me for a treatment, and as I explained how she needed to start with an internal fix to see better results, she had her own "aha" moment. She said, "I've been on Accutane, and that's just really intense on my body. And because it's taken orally, clearly something has to be going on internally to fix my skin externally. It all makes sense now! I'd rather find something that's better for me, so I need to do something inside my body to see results on the outside."

Her doctor had been trying to achieve that internal effect through Accutane, which is a naturally occurring derivative of vitamin A. But unfortunately, ingesting too much vitamin A, even though it's in a prescription form, runs the risk of causing damage to internal organs, hair loss, and severe birth defects if taken during pregnancy.

Fortunately, you can achieve the same positive results for your skin holistically (taking into consideration your entire body—physically and psychologically) and have it work just as well, if not even better! It's about making yourself healthier inside, so the outside can reap the benefits.

Here's what I suggested for my client: In addition to several topical products, such as my BORBA Age Defying Skin Lightening Spot Treatment and my BORBA Age Defying 4-in-1 Cleansing Treatment to help clear up her acne, she should include the herb milk thistle in her diet to help flush out her liver and her kidneys, as well as some of the toxins currently in her system. Because high levels of vitamin A can make your skin dry, I suggested she eat more leafy green vegetables, such as spinach, butter lettuce, and Swiss chard to help lock in moisture and aid with hydration. I also gave her instructions on how to double cleanse her skin by exfoliating first (see Chapter 3) and to make sure she used a gentle, cream-based cleanser for extra moisturization. If she implemented these small changes, both internally and externally, she would be well on her way to achieving the clear skin she desired. Just as expected, within a week she started seeing a remarkable difference.

My friend and colleague, Amy Goodman, author of *Wear This, Toss That!*, shares my philosophy and is also a firm believer in striking a balance between our external and internal environments in order to be the healthiest we can be. She says, "In our constant juggle in life, we rarely reach a homeostatic state physiologically and mentally. We eat poorly. We drink poorly. We're extremely tough on ourselves. We run ragged and take for granted that our skin will hang in there—even if genes and environmental factors like the big, bright sun are against us. But, if for a moment, we can stop and take heed and reverse bad habits, our bodies, and its largest organ—our skin—will reward us." And that's exactly what this book will help you do.

While we're often encouraged to keep our hearts, lungs, and brains healthy, we don't often think of skin as a body organ, yet it is the largest in our human system, measuring approximately 3,000 inches in the average person and weighing more than the brain. Taking care of our skin, which provides many imperative functions, such as protection, temperature control, sensory experience, and other primary tasks, is not just a beauty issue but a health issue as well. When we treat this amazing multitasker with the respect and care it deserves, we reap the benefits.

This program works for people of all skin types, ages, races, and backgrounds. A lot of people think that because they have certain hereditary challenges or issues, such as acne-prone skin, oily skin, sagging skin, or aging skin, that they'll never be able to have beautiful skin. You might be one of them; you might think that just because your mom or your grandma has a certain skin problem that you're going to have it too, and you can't do anything about it. That is completely FALSE! No, you can't change your DNA, but you can affect your body so that it triggers certain mechanisms that will make your skin and body healthier. You can start right now, and this book will help guide you through the process.

So now that you've identified what you want, what's next? You need to identify what you need most from any beauty system and figure out how it fits into your budget. Many people think they need to buy every product in a beauty line to get the desired result. But that's not necessary, even though that's how every company sells it. You'll still see a change in your skin even if you only do one thing different in your beauty routine. Small changes can have big effects!

Whether you have $10 or $1,000 to spend on your beauty regimen, you should do the same thing: identify your priorities based on what you really want and proceed based on how much you have in your budget. You can always begin by picking an inexpensive product or the least expensive product in the line and use that first to jump-start your journey toward beautiful skin. For example, if you're on a budget and your biggest problem is aging skin, start with the number one product that will give you the best benefits, which in this case is a high-level SPF product with antiaging ingredients (we'll dive into this in greater detail in Chapter 2). I wouldn't tell you to buy a serum, cleanser, or anything else. I would tell you to buy the best sunscreen for your skin type—the higher the SPF, the better (such as my BORBA Age Defying Super Crème Day Moisture SPF 100+). On top of that, you can supplement with items you can buy at the grocery store, like fish to get the benefits of omega-3 oils (see Chapter 4). It's simply a matter of putting your money into different products at the market that can benefit your skin depending on your specific condition versus spending all your money just on beauty products.

Starting with Chapter 1, you'll learn how to map out your most prominent skin challenges. I'll show you how to tackle your skin issues one at a time for the treatment of your skin and your body.

Are you ready for this challenge? You bet you are! Start by taking a picture of yourself so you can document your own before and after. It's also a good idea to ask someone, such as a close friend, spouse, or housemate, to go through this process with you. When you have a partner, she or he can help you more objectively recognize the changes you are going through. This is because you see yourself in the mirror every day and may not notice the small differences that start to add up. For instance, when I was going through my process and changing my skin, I didn't notice it as much as other people did because I was staring at a mirror every day and not seeing the bigger picture. When other people saw me going through this process, they kept telling me I looked so much better than I did the week or month before. That's when I realized it must be working!

If you don't have a partner, that's okay too. Just be patient with yourself and trust that this process is working, and that in time, the changes will become apparent to you as well as to those around you. You can also try taking your own picture each week to check on your progress.

It's time for your reinvention to begin! So take a picture, grab a partner if you have one, and let's get started.

Getting Up Close and Personal with Your Skin

EVERYONE'S SKIN IS DIFFERENT with its own unique challenges—you just need to figure out what yours are and use that as a jumping-off point on your journey. Along the way, I'll be your guide to help you assess your individual skin type and dissect the nagging problems that come with it. Just remember to be honest with yourself and really decide what changes you want to make on the outside, and together we'll make that happen from the inside out.

The average person usually has a handful of different issues with their skin. The first step is to make a list of all of your issues and then decide which change would yield the biggest benefit and begin there. For example, if you have both acne and aging skin, you need to decide what your number one concern is and move in that direction first. If it's aging, then begin with that and move to acne later. For each problem, you can start over at the beginning of this book and go through it chapter by chapter for the next skin issue you have. It's a process, but trust me—it works!

What's My Skin Type?

Most problem skin falls into five major categories: acne-prone skin, sensitive skin, aging skin, cellulite, and skin in transition. They each come with their own set of issues, challenges, and obstacles, but none are so big they can't be conquered. I'll start by breaking down each category with a simple explanation so you'll have a better idea of which ones you're facing.

Acne-prone Skin

Everyone's definition of acne is a little bit different. For most people acne means unsightly pimples, blackheads, or whiteheads on their face, chest, and/or back, which are caused when pores become clogged with bacteria, oil (sebum), and dead skin cells. Blackheads are follicles that are filled with keratin and modified sebum, an oily secretion that darkens when it oxidizes, causing the dark black color. In contrast, a whitehead is a follicle that is filled with the same material—sebum—but lacks a

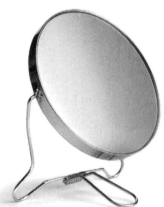

microscopic opening to the skin surface. Since the air cannot reach the follicle, the material is not oxidized and thus remains white. Typically you can get rid of whiteheads much quicker than blackheads.

Acne can also be open papules, inflamed red bumps without a head (like a whitehead), or pustules, which contain pus, oil, and dead skin cells. Pustules can also appear as red circles with a white or yellow center.

A more serious type of acne is cystic acne, which consists of bumps filled with pus that are often five millimeters or more in diameter across. This condition can often be very painful and cannot be cured overnight. Acne can also manifest as rosacea, which is characterized by skin that is easily subjected to blushing (resulting from small, dilated blood vessels beneath the surface), redness, or swelling, or it can be a pattern of broken blood vessels with a weblike appearance. Things like environment, climate changes, and stress hormones can also be triggers for acne.

Sensitive Skin

Sensitive skin can range from someone who blushes easily to someone who breaks out when their skin touches another person. Maybe you're allergic to many ingredients in skin-care products, or maybe your skin gets overly dry or oily because of the products you use. Psoriasis is another condition which is characterized by raised red patches or bumps appearing on any part of your body. These all fall under the sensitive-skin umbrella. Bacteria, environment, skin-care products, changes in temperature, and interpersonal contact are all triggers for people with sensitive skin.

Aging Skin

Aging skin is characterized by texture in the form of little lines, deep wrinkles, or furrow marks; it is also often crepey or sagging. It can also be characterized by a loss of radiance and a general dullness in your epidermis. The passage of time and not taking proper care of your skin as you age are the major causes of aging skin.

Cellulite

Cellulite is defined as that less-than-desirable dimpled appearance of the skin that can show up on your thighs, hips, or buttocks—similar to cottage cheese or an orange peel. It's caused by the distortion of fat deposits in the connective tissue beneath the skin, which can change its outer texture.

Cellulite is genetic, but it's also caused by poor circulation throughout the body and skin. Due to certain hormonal factors, women are far more likely to get cellulite than men. In fact, men rarely develop cellulite. The influences of genetic factors have not been investigated fully, but any bit of genetic predisposition may make you more likely to develop cellulite. So if the genes you inherited from your mother or grandmother make you a likely candidate, it would be in your best interest to live a lifestyle that will prevent cellulite as much as possible.

It's also important to know that this condition can improve or worsen depending on what you eat to help fortify collagen production in your epidermis. Exercise can also help by smoothing out the memory of the skin. (And, yes, your skin does have memory.) Research shows that long after you do anything to alter the state of your skin, it can become hypersensitive in the location you worked on and will "remember" the new and improved condition you created days, weeks, or even months later.

Skin in Transition

As you go from one stage of life to another, your skin also goes through transition and change. For example, pregnancy alters not just your body shape but your skin as well. Losing or gaining weight can cause your skin to transform. Going from your teens into your twenties is a transition. Moving from your twenties into your thirties and from your thirties into your forties and so on is a transition. Entering perimenopause and menopause are big ones, and when you hit sixty, there is some serious work you need to do with your skin. The bottom line is that as you move into any new stage of your life, there's a good chance your skin will experience a change as well, and knowing how to treat it is the key to keeping it healthy.

Let's Map It Out

Mapping or analyzing your skin isn't just for your face. It can also be done over your entire body. Skin challenges can crop up anywhere, but right now, let's focus on your fabulous, fixable face and see what needs a change.

By examining the sketch below and recognizing where your issues are, you'll be able to dramatically enhance the effectiveness of every treatment you choose and make your own prescription for a home-care regimen completely focused on your unique needs.

This map divides the face into nine distinct zones, each with its own set of potential problems and individual skin concerns. Read through these descriptions. Do they sound like things you might be doing? Take a look in the mirror and consider each area where your challenges are popping up, and get ready to start solving them one problem zone at a time.

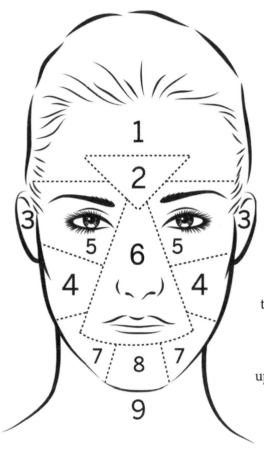

Figure 1. Face Zone Map

Zone 1

Skin challenges in this prominent area could be cropping up from things you're doing and using every day. It's all about taking care of your skin the right way, so if you're not properly removing your makeup or facial and hair products from the sides of your forehead, that could be what's clogging your pores and causing breakouts. In addition, some of your beauty products themselves may actually contain ingredients that are creating irritation. According to reflexology, biologically these two zones are connected to your bladder and digestive system, so if these areas are dried out, possible causes may be not hydrating enough throughout your day or not completely getting rid of all the toxins that enter your system daily. Make sure you drink at least 64 ounces of water a day (and see Chapter 8 for a great seven-day detox)!

Zone 2

If you're having trouble in the middle of your forehead, try looking at what you're eating and drinking when you're kicking back and having a night on the town. Because this area is connected to your liver, those pesky lines and pimples that keep popping up might be indicative of too much alcohol, midnight snacking, or dining on food that is delicious but far too rich for your system. Trouble on your bothersome brow could also be caused by age or lack of proper moisturizing. (Check out Chapter 2 to find products that can help alleviate some of these problems.)

Zone 3

Are your ears burning? It's probably not because someone is talking about you, but may actually be a sign that your kidneys are in need of some TLC. They might be troubled due to an influx of too much salt, red meat, and caffeine. So make sure you drink lots of water to help detox your system, and see Chapter 4 for some other helpful culinary suggestions. Age could be a factor, or even too much exposure to the sun (see Chapter 6 for solutions). Redness in this area could also be a symptom of over-touching your lobes or even stress (Chapter 3 has some great stress-relieving tips).

Zone 4

Take a look at the apples of your cheeks. If you're seeing clogged pores or even broken capillaries, it could be connected to allergies, pollution, or smoking. Improper cleansing, excess sweating, or even using makeup with the wrong ingredients could also be culprits (see Chapter 2 to learn about the best makeup for your skin type and Chapter 3 for how to properly exfoliate your face).

Zone 5

If you see those oh-so-unpopular dark circles under your eyes (most of us have them!) or even bumps and clogged pores around the eye orbit right under the surface, it might be time to reevaluate your daily routine. Yes, those circles can be hereditary, but they can also be exacerbated by not catching enough z's, not getting rid of the toxins in your body properly, allergies, or even a diet that's lacking essential nutritional elements or water. (See Chapter 4 for a list of foods that you can add to your diet and Chapter 7 for some easy suggestions to help eradicate the darkness.)

Zone 6

Your nose always knows what's up and can tell you a lot about what's happening on your inside. If you tend to get a red nose, it may be indicative of blood pressure that's higher than it should be or even too much internal emotional stress. Breakouts, discoloration, or an unwanted mustache might be telling you that you have a hormone imbalance (see Chapters 6 and 7 for suggestions). And if you find yourself with irritation around your lip line, check out the ingredients in your lipstick, lip balm, or lip liners. They may actually contain possible acne-inducing ingredients! (See Chapter 2 for some guidance on choosing products containing helpful actives for these issues.)

Zone 7

Breakouts and clogged pores along both sides of your jawbone near your ears could be caused by anything, ranging from a hormonal imbalance to improper exfoliation, or may even be linked to dental issues. So if you're having trouble with your choppers, gums, or even wisdom teeth, they might actually be the culprit. (Check out Chapter 4 for a list of foods that can help and Chapter 7 for suggestions on how to abolish acne.)

Zone 8

If the center of your chin is causing you grief, it might be connected to problems in your small intestine. Digestion issues or food allergies could actually be linked to your breakouts. Try eliminating certain trigger foods one by one to find out what might be causing a breakout (see Chapter 4 for some food alternatives that might help). These breakouts may also be the result of a hormonal imbalance (Chapters 2, 3, and 4 have some great tips to help) or even using skin-care products that are irritating your skin (see Chapter 2 for a list of ingredients you can use to eradicate breakouts).

Zone 9

Your neck and chest can suffer from the same types of skin challenges as your face. If you find that these areas are sensitive or irritated, it could possibly be a reaction to the fragrances in the products you're using, including lotions and perfumes. It can also be the result of too much stress (see Chapter 3 for some helpful hints). Those lines, grooves, or discoloration come with aging, but fortunately, Chapters 2, 4, 5, 6, and 7 are full of ideas on how to help decrease the appearance of these conditions.

Now that you have your picture and you know what your most challenging problem is, it's time to start making your changes.

Fixing Things in a Jiffy or Taking Your Time

When it comes to skin problems, it's important to realize that there are challenges that can be solved quickly and others that may take more time. It will work best for you if you can identify which of your issues falls into which category and know ahead of time how long each will take to resolve so frustration doesn't set in. For example, toning a jiggly waistline is going to take longer to fix than smoothing out the lines and wrinkles in your face. Smaller areas of your epidermis, like your face or your hands and areas that are thinner, can react a little bit faster to treatment than the thicker parts of your skin. So having a list of these things and an understanding of how long each one will take will help decrease any major aggravation on your part.

While skin concerns typically fall into the categories of either quick fixes or long fixes, the greater the effort, the faster and more complete the resolution. But if you have an important event coming up, there is a program that many Hollywood A-listers use to get red-carpet ready in just seven days. (See Chapter 8.)

Quicker fixes include conditions such as:

- Mild acne
- Fine lines and wrinkles
- Aging of the face
- Aging of the hands
- Stretch marks

• Improving the general tonality of the whole body

Slower fixes include conditions such as:

• Moderate, stage-three, or cystic acne (serious papules and pustules)
• Deep-furrow wrinkles
• Crepey skin
• Sagging skin
• Stretch marks
• Hyperpigmentation

There are many issues to choose from, but tackling them one by one with the right amount of patience will give you the best chance for success.

The Proof Is in the Prevention

You're doing all this work right now to identify your major skin problems, so it's really important to absorb all of the knowledge about how to fix them so you'll be able to prevent the same issues from happening again. Use this book as your cheat sheet in the future. Once you've succeeded in your goal, you can use this plan as a reference to keep you on track.

As you begin your journey, the biggest thing to know is that even if you start to revert to your old habits, you can quickly make up for lost time and get back on track, so don't give up. And yes, new and different problems will continually arise throughout your life as you age, so it's just as important to start preventing other skin concerns that may pop up as you go through transitions in your life as it is to know how to fix your current issues. The better equipped you are for future challenges, the easier it will be to stop them before they get out of hand.

Be In Tune with Your Body

In general, the most important thing I can tell you is to really listen to your body when it comes to skin care. You might experience a tingle in your skin that lets you know a blemish is going to come on. You can feel it. So start treating it before it turns into a problem. Don't wait. If you know that your mother, grandmother, and father all got dark circles under their eyes as they aged, you know that you need to start working on preventing that condition now. The key is to be in tune with the song your body is singing in terms of what it wants and what it needs.

If your body is telling you it's hungry or thirsty, then you need to feed it or hydrate it, because when you do that properly, your body is going to produce the chemicals, collagen, and synapses that will synergize your body from the inside out. The end result will make you healthier—and you'll look better. It's a simple concept, and if you do it correctly, you'll be able to stop skin issues before they happen and quickly take care of the ones that do happen.

2

Turning Your Beauty Routine Inside Out

NOW THAT YOU'VE SELECTED your troublesome skin issues, it's time to get started. The first step is to investigate your products to figure out which ingredients are helping and which might actually be hindering you in your quest for clearer skin. From there, we'll explore your options for repair, beginning with the products you may already have but never thought of using for your specific skin challenge. We're going to get creative, innovative, and downright investigative. Let's begin!

What's in Your Products?

It's time to take a look inside your drawers, cabinets, and shelves and examine the products you already own to identify ingredients that can help you with your current skin challenge. You might be surprised by the things that turn out to be the most beneficial for you.

Instead of racing out to buy a bunch of expensive products that are specific to your skin problems, you might already have products in your home—originally intended for another skin issue—that you can use that contain the same active ingredients you need for your current skin concern. For example, in most antiaging products, the active ingredient that treats deep wrinkles is retinol, which is actually even more effective for acne. Retinol is added to antiaging products because of its moisturizing properties. So if you have acne, try using any light-based, antiaging items (closer in consistency to a lotion rather than a heavy, thick cream), because they might be even more effective and gentler on your skin than your traditional antiacne items.

In general, it's good to keep your skin-care products for about two years (unless the label says otherwise), even if you don't use them. This is because your skin changes a lot over the course of a year due to factors such as weather, travel, and hormone fluctuations. So if you buy something that isn't working for you right now, keep it because it might help with a future skin-care challenge.

Be sure to keep in mind that every person's skin is unique. So while I am suggesting specific ingredients that help

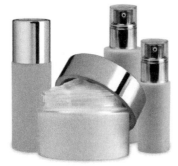

with various skin-care challenges, you should also consult your own skin esthetician, doctor, or dermatologist to make sure you are using products with the correct percentages of ingredients for your body. While a high percentage of an ingredient may work well for one person, it may be too strong for someone with sensitive skin, for example. Therefore, before using a new product, be sure to ask an expert to help you design a personalized regimen for your specific challenge with the ingredients I suggest.

The ingredients I mention are based on their widespread availability in the United States. Most of them are available in the products sold at your local stores or markets, as well as online. These aren't hard-to-find ingredients that are specific to high-end products.

Before we get started, here are a few rules of thumb: First, if you're using an ingredient in a topical skin-care product, try to ingest foods and drinks that contain that same ingredient because it will maximize the synergy within your system and help you obtain optimum benefits for your skin. For example, if you eat foods containing omega-3, 6, and 9, like avocados, fish, and wheat germ oil, and also use products infused with omega-3, 6, and 9 (or even use avocados topically in a mask), that will be incredibly powerful in reducing inflammation in your body and helping to nourish your skin, making it look more youthful. Another example is to eat and drink foods rich in vitamin C, like fruits, berries, and orange juice, while also using topical products containing vitamin C. This is an excellent combination for giving skin strength and combating free-radical damage in acne-prone, aging, and sensitive skin.

The second rule of thumb is to use the right amount of your products. Here is a basic rundown of the amount of each type of product you should be using during application: For cleansers, I recommend using a quarter-sized amount at the minimum to properly clean your skin. And for a double cleanse, you'll need a quarter-sized amount of your exfoliator and a quarter-sized amount of your secondary cleanser. For serums (or concentrates or treatments), you only need to use a nickel-sized amount. For your nighttime facial moisturizers, you should use a dime-sized amount.

All for One: Ingredient Basics

The top nutritional ingredients in beauty supplements typically consist of common vitamins your body needs, such as A, C, and E, as well as some not-so-obvious ingredients like natural botanical extracts with antioxidants that fight free-radical attacks, amino acids that can help boost your skin's collagen levels, and proteins that can replace the proteins that break down in your skin.

It's also important to note that a lot of products have many ingredients that work for several skin types across the board. You can find alpha hydroxy acid (AHA) and beta hydroxy acid (BHA), such as salicylic acid, retinol, and glycolic acid, in a number of different skin-care products. The key is to find the right percentage content for your skin type. The actives, or ingredients with the higher percentages, are listed at the top of the ingredient list on every label. So when buying a new product, check out the label first to make sure it has a good amount of the active you're looking for, as advised by your esthetician or doctor.

So how can two skin types use the same product? Here is an example. Let's say a woman has a daughter who is using a mass-market acne cleanser containing 2.5 percent salicylic acid to get rid of her breakouts. The mom can actually use that same cleanser by mixing it with a little bit of her antiaging cream or another cleansing cream that's a little thicker and more moisturizing and she will get a deeper effect of her antiaging product. This is because the same ingredient of salicylic acid with exfoliating beads is going to help prepare her skin a lot better than traditional anti-aging products alone. The added element from the acne cleanser can improve the effectiveness of her antiaging cream.

It also works in reverse. The daughter can use a light antiaging lotion to help with her acne. The amount of retinol contained in the antiaging formula is going to be more effective and even gentler on the daughter's acne than some of the traditional antiacne products. It's both beneficial and cost-effective to share products in your home that contain the same essential ingredients.

If you're younger and have a T-zone area with dry skin and you want to spot treat that, and your mother is looking for a moisturizer for her aging skin, you can both share shea butter cream (or even a soy or vitamin E- or C-based moisturizer) specifically formulated for the face for both skin types. And in the shower, you can both use a cream-based cleanser for antiaging to get the effects of the retinol—you for your acne and your mom for her aging concerns.

Your Product Lineup

Now it's time to take out all your products, line them up, and group them by the product benefits. Separate everything by what you use it for: cleansers, moisturizers, problem treatment items, sunscreens, bronzers, and whatever else you have. Then within each category, arrange them according to the ingredients that help with acne, antiaging, firming the skin, or whatever it is (see details below). Then you can mix and match how you use them based on how your skin changes over the month. Hormones may cause you to break out or get dry patches. A stressful situation may cause your skin to become oilier. Whatever the case, your skin can be unpredictable, but having different products on hand for different conditions that might arise is extremely helpful.

Let's start with the basics. Determine the skin challenge you presently have, go to the section that follows to see what ingredients you should look for, and work on that issue first. Then, when a new challenge arises, return to this chapter, look for those ingredients, and fix that problem next. Having a variety of products on hand will allow you to search for the new ingredients in your own cabinets before you head out to the store to make a purchase.

So what ingredients should you look for? Each skin type has its own list of what can help, so I'll break it down for you below. When you're done reading, you can start building your own skin-care system with the ingredients you already have and supplement what you're missing by purchasing a few new products if necessary.

Key Ingredients for Acne

If you have acne, products containing sulfur should be at the top of your priority list. Sulfur absorbs quickly into the skin and won't cause any irritation or redness. It usually works as fast, if not faster, than other more common antiacne ingredients. Sulfur is also great because it layers with makeup, moisturizers, and pretty much anything else you put on top of it without any peeling. In general, products with 4–8 percent sulfur are the best for most acne-prone skin. Lactic acid, malic acid, and mandelic acid are also effective ingredients, so look for those at the top of the ingredient list too. Salicylic acid will also work, but it can cause redness in some people.

Benzoyl peroxide, which helps remove bacteria in the follicles and reduces whiteheads and blackheads, is another common element to look for. You can also look for products containing isotretinoin, which helps to reduce oil production, soothes the inflammation caused by pimples, cysts, and pustules, and can also help unblock clogged pores.

If you're going holistic, ingredients such as oatmeal and comfrey root have amazingly soothing properties. You should also look for products that contain polyphenols, such as pomegranate, which is a great anti-inflammatory agent. In addition, find products containing

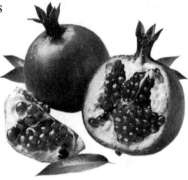

natural exfoliants, such as apricot seeds, olive seeds, light walnut husks, or any type of jojoba beads, which can all help loosen and lift away dead skin cells to reveal smoother, softer, and radiant new skin.

Key Ingredients for Antiaging

In addition to common ingredients like vitamins A, C, and E, alpha hydroxy acid, and glycolic acid, the number one ingredient to look for in an antiaging product is hyaluronic acid—the higher the percentage the better. I always suggest to my clients that they begin with a lower percentage and then go higher, depending on how his or her body reacts and absorbs the product. (You should consult your esthetician or doctor to figure out the right percentage for your skin type.) Coming in at a close second is retinol, which is a pure form of vitamin A, so look for that to be one of the first ingredients on the label. Retinol is the key to accelerating cell turnover so healthier cells rejuvenate faster, making your skin look smoother and younger. Also look for any ingredient with a "tide" in it, like tripeptides and hepapeptides, as well as palmitates. These will all help improve your skin's appearance and assist in the regeneration of the skin's collagen levels.

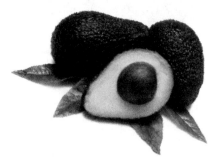

You also want to find products with quality oils that combat wrinkles, like avocado oil, aloe, cocoa butter, or safflower seed oil, which is a natural and lightweight hydrating oil that helps to moisturize, nourish, and restructure the skin. Other helpful ingredients include glycerin, ascorbic acid, and specific binders like vitamin E, which is excellent for moisture retention and helping the skin breathe. Last, green tea extract is an excellent ingredient due to its anti-inflammatory properties, and it can reduce the appearance of puffiness, wrinkles, fine lines, and large pores.

For those pesky crow's feet, try products that include hyaluronic acid and glow-enhancing argan oil to provide you with a solid moisturizing base. These are both common ingredients that can be found in many inexpensive products sold at your local drugstore.

Key Ingredients for Sensitive Skin

If you have sensitive skin, you should limit the amount of chemical actives in any creams, lotions, gels, or liquids you use and instead look for naturally derived ingredients that help coat your skin and protect it against the harsh elements in your environment. The more natural a product you can get, the less potential irritation you'll experience. This also means you should try to avoid products with added fragrance (items scented by the actual oils themselves should be okay). Just be aware that some people with sensitive skin might not be able to tolerate many of the natural ingredients as well, so consult with your esthetician, primary care physician, or dermatologist to make sure the products you choose are safe to use on your skin. But in general, concentrate on finding products that have a good dimethicone barrier (an ingredient that helps to repair or heal damaged skin); these include protective silicones, titanium dioxide, or zinc oxide. Make sure there is anywhere from 2–5 percent of whichever of these ingredients you choose in your products.

Look for natural elements that will soothe your skin with anti-inflammatory agents, such as olive oil, oat kernel extract, chamomile, papaya, and grape seed oil. Other ingredients to look for include colloidal oatmeal (refined) and glycerin (a luscious hydrator that allows the skin to breathe), which can both soothe the skin and even out skin tone. In addition, both aloe vera and sulfur can help treat chronic redness and inflammation.

One last ingredient that I love, but that isn't found in a lot of products, is the spice turmeric. It's incredible for sensitive skin and has very potent antioxidant and anti-inflammatory properties.

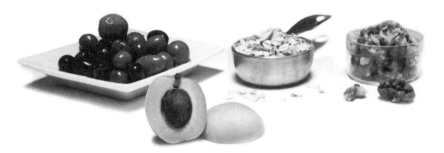

Key Ingredients for Cellulite

Retinol A and caffeine (in gel or cream form) are great for battling cellulite. As discussed, retinol A moisturizes the skin and can soften the underlying tissues that may be causing the problem. Caffeine can help loosen and carry away any fat that is being stored and trapped under your skin. Other ingredients with those same antioxidant and collagen-building effects include aminophylline and theophylline, as well as creams containing vitamins A, E, and C.

You can also look for certain seed extracts like gotu kola, which can fortify collagen and improve the body's circulation, or grape seed extract, which has antioxidant properties that can help the skin fight free radicals. Aescin is another great ingredient because it helps seal the walls of capillaries on the skin and also improves blood flow. Rounding out the list of holistic ingredients to look for are milk and almond oil, which can help create a smoother skin tone.

Key Ingredients for Skin in Transition

Because a woman's skin changes throughout the various stages of her life—from pregnancy and decade changes to perimenopause and menopause—you should be looking for items containing the herb black cohosh across the board. (Black cohosh can also be purchased as a stand-alone oral supplement in vitamin stores.) Using black cohosh both internally and externally will help you balance your hormone levels and provide relief for your skin (and your emotions). It will fortify your skin with some of those same ingredients you're going to be putting into your body.

When faced with skin in transition, your best approach is to figure out which products work the best overall on your body and not waste a ton of money on several different products that may not work together. My advice is to literally test the areas of your skin where you're having the challenges with different products, and when you find one that works, use it as a single product on your face and body versus having multiple products on different parts of your skin. So many women make the mistake of doing that. They will put antiacne products on certain areas of their skin, antiaging products around their eye and deep-wrinkle area, and moisturizer on other parts of their face. And surprisingly, that isn't going to give you the most beneficial results. Instead, use just that one product all over and you'll start to see an improvement.

If you're trying to get rid of stretch marks, look for products with the highest percentages of salicylic acid that you can find. Salicylic acid is phenomenally helpful in breaking down the proteins that hold the dead skin cells together. Cholic acid is also great for stretch marks because it contains emulsifying properties that help break down fat cell walls. Soybean is another helpful ingredient for camouflaging and evening out skin tone. You should also use products that contain cocoa butter for mild stretch marks or Retin-A for more severe ones.

Cucumber extract is not only great for soothing and relieving dry and puffy skin, its antioxidant and moisturizing properties help revitalize skin. In addition, shea butter contains a lot of vitamin E and is extremely nourishing for skin with stretch marks. You can use it as a stand-alone item or look for it in the list of ingredients in any product at the store. Suntan lotion (even when you're not out in the sun) has a lot of oils in it, and it's great for reducing the appearance of stretch marks. After you exfoliate in the shower, dry off and then rub on a thin layer of suntan lotion on your skin—enough so it absorbs into your skin, but not a greasy coat like you would apply when going to the beach. When you do go to the beach, make sure you cover up your body so that it doesn't get exposed to the sun, because stretch marks may turn darker with sun exposure due to their pigment content. Retinyl palmitate is also great for firming the skin; look for more than 2 percent retinyl palmitate on the label—anything less than that won't be as effective.

Key Ingredients for Combination Skin

When dealing with combination skin, you may need to treat individual areas of your skin differently than other areas, which is a slight variance from the treatment of skin in transition, where you're looking for one overall product. If you find yourself with several challenges all at once, read back through this section and mix and match the products you are looking for depending on which skin challenge you're treating. You might need one product for the breakouts on your forehead and another to treat your dry jawline. Experiment to find the right combination of elements that will work for your individual skin concerns.

Delivery System

Now that you know what the best products are for your skin problem, make sure they come in the right types of containers or packaging. I'm not recommending that you go out and buy the latest technology for product dispensing, but you should try to find products that provide a combination of natural and chemical activation when applied. That means you want items you will actually manually massage into your skin to allow the products to penetrate more effectively.

When it comes to products other than your cleansers, which are pretty stable, you should look for skin-care items with pumps or in airtight containers. Over time, oxygen will denigrate the activity level of whatever formulation is inside, so it's important that you try to pump your products versus squeezing them for maximum activity. However, the exception is for your treatment products, which include serums and any problem-specific solution products with actives designed to spot treat your challenge (as opposed to a more general moisturizer or cleanser). Look for those in a bottle instead, preferably a dark-colored one, to help minimize exposure to light.

3

The Dirty Dozen:
The Hidden Skin Saboteurs
in Your Daily Life

NOW THAT YOU'VE selected the troublesome issues you want to fix, it's time to turn your attention to other things that people often overlook when it comes to their skin. This chapter will give you surprising facts about how everyday items and everyday habits may be hurting your skin. The way you exfoliate, the tools you use to clean your skin, and even your stress level can all have a direct impact on some of your current skin challenges. Fortunately, there are easy fixes to most of these problems.

Top Twelve Secret Skin Shockers

Let's start by taking a look at what you've been using to apply or remove your makeup, foundation, and lotions. Did you ever stop to think these items might be causing some of the skin challenges you've been experiencing? It is likely that somewhere between your brushes, sponges, and cotton swabs, your skin has been trying to tell you it's had enough and wants you to clean up your act! By making just a few small adjustments, you can make that happen.

1. Bacteria-bearing Brushes

When it comes to makeup brushes, a thorough sanitizing every three uses is necessary to clean away the dirt and oils that have saturated the bristles. In addition, makeup brushes should be replaced every six months. If you don't disinfect the brushes after every use or few uses and you're using them all over your face repeatedly, they can easily transfer bacteria back and forth from your brush to your makeup and back

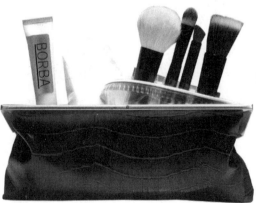

onto your skin. The hair on the brushes, if it's natural hair from an animal, will literally, just like your own hair, saturate with bacteria that will then saturate into the actual follicle itself. Natural hair absorbs more bacteria than synthetic hair because it's pure keratin, and synthetic hair has bristles that are more solid, so you have a better chance of disinfecting a synthetic brush than one made from natural hair. However, regardless of which one you use, even though you are cleaning the brushes, the process will still never completely eliminate all of the bacteria, and it will continue to deposit small amounts onto your skin with each use. This causes free-radical damage, which can then create some of your skin challenges, like acne, premature aging, or sagging (crepey) skin. To avoid this cycle, find an affordable set of brushes that will allow you to replace them every six months without breaking your bank account.

It's also best to use a natural-based cleaning product to wash your brushes. The BORBA line includes a mangosteen spray (the BORBA Atomizer) that can be used for this purpose. There are alternatives, of course. You can clean the bristles of your brushes with any sort of antibacterial liquid, such as a hand sanitizer, or with anything moisturizing or infused with vitamin E. (Be careful: using a product with a high alcohol content may actually break down the bristles of both synthetic and natural brushes.) You can make your own solution as well. Simply mix two drops of tea tree oil in one-eighth cup of hot water and pour into a small spray bottle. Mist your brushes with this mix every day before you use them (and still give them a thorough cleaning every three

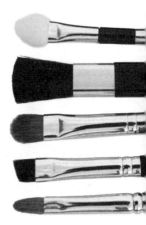

days). Wipe down the brushes with a clean washcloth or towel until there is no excess powder or liquid left on the bristles; then do your makeup application. This is the best way to help reduce the bacteria from the bristles and minimize the transfer of bacteria. If you keep the solution in a cool, dry place (like under your sink in the bathroom), it should be good for about two weeks before you need to make a new batch.

2. Suspect Sponges

If you have a choice between using a sponge or your fingers to apply your makeup, sponges are better, because fingers that haven't been properly cleansed with good old-fashioned soap and water can transfer bacteria, oils, and other free radicals a lot quicker than sponges will (and even if you've cleansed your hands, a sponge is still best in my opinion). Unless you use your index finger, you're most likely going to be pulling and tugging on your skin worse than you would using a sponge. I don't care how clean you think your fingers are, they will still have bacteria on them, which will be transferred to your skin. And that same bacteria will then be put back into the product you are dipping your fingers into during application. On the pro-sponge side, the sponges you buy are actually closed-sealed in a production process that has to be completely sterile, as opposed to the skin on your fingers, which will most likely never be completely sterile. So if you're using a sponge right out of the package and dipping it right into your products, both will be clean, thereby greatly reducing the transfer of bacteria.

When it comes to those square sponges that have six different sides or ones that are triangular shaped, a lot of women make a very common mistake and use that same darn square over and over until all of the "clean" sides are used up. They'll continue to dip it back into their concealer pot every day until all the surfaces are utilized. But the truth is, after you use the sponge once, by the next time you go to use another side for an application, the formulation and the bacteria have already leaked through and tainted the other surface you haven't used yet. So you need to throw it away as soon as you're done using it once to avoid recontaminating your skin. And for the record, you *cannot* wash the sponges with soap and water for reuse when you're done. If you do that, because they're already harboring all that bacteria, letting the sponges air dry will only manifest even more germs and bacteria, which will continue to grow. Don't do it! But if you're concerned about using so many sponges each week, take a pair of scissors cleaned with alcohol and cut the sponges in half. That way you'll get twice the number of sponges and won't have to buy them as often.

To Share or Not to Share?

It's very important to avoid sharing personal-hygiene products. Acne, as well as other skin issues, can spread quickly if items such as towels, makeup sponges, or brushes are used by more than one person. I always remind my clients that sharing cosmetics and other products that touch your skin is a big NO-NO!

Here's why: Your skin secretes sebum, which is an oily substance that helps keep skin soft and water-resistant. Every time you wipe your skin against something, a mixture of sebum, dead skin cells, and dirt is transferred to that surface. Imagine using someone else's brush or towel: If some of his or her debris comes into contact with one of your pores or hair follicles, you may wind up with an infected pore or follicle that results in a nasty-looking pustule or zit. Of course, you only want clean items to come into contact with your skin in the first place, but when you add another person's sebum concoction to the mix, it's like gambling with your pores, and the odds are not in your favor.

To avoid this problem, many of my celebrity clients simply bring their own set of brushes and sponges to the set every day, taking full responsibility for the cleanliness of their skin. So always be sure to use your own brushes and sponges, don't lend them out, and keep them clean!

3. Lose the Loofah

Let's move on to what you may be using to clean your skin: loofahs and sponges. A lot of my clients use loofahs; others just love those sea-foam sponges and will use them virtually forever. But really, the truth of the matter is you should use a new loofah or sponge every week and toss the old one. Some discount stores carry loofahs in bulk. You can buy a bunch of them for as little as a quarter apiece in some places. At that price, that's just a dollar a month. And it is so worth it!

Here's why it's so important not to use and reuse your loofah over and over again. Because of its intricate webbing, a wet loofah will literally pick up dirt and debris from your skin and keep it locked inside. If you've ever had a scab, dead skin, or excess skin on your feet from wearing high heels or sandals, those will be left in your loofah after scrubbing. Sometimes you can actually see the debris in the webbing. Even if you try to rinse it away, you will never clean it out completely, and every time you wash, you will be adding that bacteria back onto your body. And as you know, that's never a good thing.

It's best to have several loofahs on hand to rotate, but just know that you can also wash a loofah in scalding hot water for at least 10–15 seconds and that should kill the majority of the bacteria (not all, but most). You can also toss your loofah into the washing machine and that should do the trick as well (and no, the fibers won't break down during the cycle).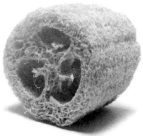

I suggest you purchase the type of loofah that resembles a washcloth. They are as effective as the big poofie loofahs, but they can be washed in your washing machine as often as you'd like. The washing machine washes out all of the dirt and debris, and the heat of the dryer will kill any remaining bacteria. One of these loofah cloths is probably about a ten-dollar investment, but it should last for six months to a year when it is properly cared for.

Using one of these cloths will also help you massage in the actives you're putting on your skin, body, and even your face. It will slough away dead skin cells and make your skin more absorbent so you can maximize the product's benefits. It's a multipurpose purchase!

And if you're wondering about washcloths, in my opinion, it's still better to use a loofah, because washcloths can be more abrasive and don't slough off as much dead skin on your body as loofahs do. In addition, a loofah only needs about one-quarter the amount of product that a washcloth needs to give you benefits.

4. Towel Tricks

When you come out of the shower, you feel clean, but a lot of times you get the remaining excess oil and dirt off your skin with your towel. Unfortunately, the next time you go to dry off, that

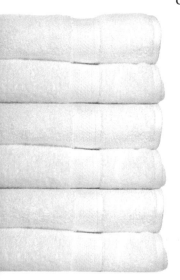

old oil and dirt will transfer right back onto your skin. So it's really important to wash your towels at least once or twice a week.

I totally respect anyone who is eco-friendly and doesn't want to continually wash their towels and waste water. So if you are going to use your towel for multiple days, here's a suggestion: use it in quadrants, meaning if you have a long bath towel, use it quarter sections at a time. Then you should put it in the laundry after you've used each of the sections. If you don't want to do that, just use smaller towels and use one side for one day and the other side the next day and then wash it, because towels harbor a tremendous amount of bacteria, oil, and dirt, and who wants to keep putting that back onto their skin every day? Not me!

You should be doing this regardless of whether or not you have problem skin. The more dirt and oil that's left on your skin, the more your pores will clog which will prevent your products from penetrating your skin.

5. Bedding

Those luxury linens you've been lounging on may be the under-lying offender creating some of your skin problems. Sheets need to be changed once a week *at a minimum* for the body to stay clear of growing bacteria from oils, sweat, and dead skin cells. If you notice that your skin continues to experience challenges, try switching detergents—that could definitely be another culprit as well. Try switching to a fragrance-free product or even one that's used for infants' clothing.

If you are a bare-naked sleeper and are single, it's best to try sleeping in different areas on your bed each night. The accumulation of sweat and oils in the sheets can give you acne on your back, and moving around can minimize that issue. If you share the bed with someone else, it's best to spray your sheets with a tea tree oil mix (just like you would make to clean your makeup brushes, but use a 10- to 12-ounce bottle of purified water and add ten drops of tea tree oil), if you're going to be using the sheets for an extended period of time (as in one or two weeks).

It's a must for your face that you change your pillowcase twice a week to avoid recycling trapped dirt, oil, and bacteria. Here is the system I suggest: Use a fresh pillowcase on the first night. The next night, flip it over and that's your "new" pillowcase; on the third night, you need to change it out with a new one, and it's a continuous cycle from there. That way, when you lay your cleansed face on the pillowcase, it will stay clean, and your clean sheets will allow your skin to breathe. It is so worth it! For oily, acne-prone, or sensitive skin, use cotton sheets, but for aging skin, silk sheets are best.

6. Couches and Other Furniture

Person-to-person contact or sharing products aren't the only methods of transferring bacteria. Furniture can also shift unwanted dirt, oil, and bacteria onto your skin. Fortunately, there are easy things you can do to help keep these culprits at bay. First, take a look at where you normally sit on your couch and then look at where your skin challenges are cropping up. If they are on the exposed parts of your body, like your arms or your back, places that most commonly come into contact with the material of your couch, you may have found one of the triggers for your skin challenge. The couch actually has a lot of oils and bacteria on it from you and the other people who sit on it, which might be the trouble-causing trigger. It builds up and stays there, so every time your skin touches that material, it further fuels the problem.

One easy and obvious solution is to make sure you have those parts of your skin covered when you sit on your couch. You can also cover your couch with a fresh throw or blanket and wash it frequently. In addition, try to have the material on your couch cleaned as often as you can, either with a topical nonstaining disinfectant spray designed for couches or at the dry cleaners if the cushions are removable. You'll notice a world of difference if you do! If you have a darker couch, you can try spraying on the tea tree oil and water mixture. However, be careful if your couch is cream or white because the oil is green in color and could stain.

By the way, bacteria also rests in common areas like the doorknobs of your bathroom, the keyboard of your computer, and on countertops. So it is very important that at least once a week you disinfect all of those surfaces to avoid any further transfer of bacteria. The less bad bacteria you have lying around your home, the less likely you are to transfer some of it onto your skin and create further problems.

Don't Overuse Antibacterial Products

Bacteria lives everywhere. You can't get away from it, and you shouldn't try. Along with the bad bacteria, there are good bacteria that our bodies need to be healthy. While it's one thing to use an antibacterial product on your hands occasionally to reduce the chance of spreading germs, doing so too often strips away some of the things that your skin needs to stay moisturized and healthy. Always be conscious of how often you're using any product, and use it only when you really need to.

7. Phones and Cell Phones

When it comes to your phone or your cell phone, it's important that you wipe it off or use an antibacterial spray to clean it as often as you can. The oils, dirt, and bacteria on your face that build up naturally every day immediately transfer onto the phone as you chat away, so when you go to use it again, they transfer right back onto your skin. So as a rule, wipe down your telephone receiver and cell phone with alcohol or a disinfectant wipe on a daily basis to avoid the continuous cycle. Of course, to minimize this problem even further, try using a speaker phone or a hands-free option as often as you can.

8. Hairy Situations

I love long hair. I think many people do, but if you do have flowing locks, here's something to consider. The more your hair touches your skin, the more it's releasing that oily sebum, which may be causing some of your challenges. It doesn't matter if your issue is breakouts, sensitive skin, or aging skin—if you have extra oil coming into contact with your epidermis, you're going to potentially have more challenges.

This is what I suggest: try to keep your hair off your face and your other problem areas as much as possible, even if it's long. Leave the curls on the side. If you have bangs, have them hit closer to your eyebrows versus your forehead if that's at all possible. The less your hair comes into contact with your skin, the better. Let that oil stay where it should and keep your locks nourished instead of becoming the catalyst for more skin issues!

And if you're suffering from scalp challenges such as acne, psoriasis, or dandruff, don't think that the more you wash it, the more dandruff you'll get. That's a myth. You should be treating your scalp every single day, because if you're not doing that, the problems are going to compile. Then at night, when you're lying on your pillow, if you're not changing out the pillowcase, the problems will compound, thereby causing more challenges for your skin.

The solution is simple. Take care of your scalp on a daily basis until the issue subsides, keep the contact your hair has with your face and back to a minimum, and try to avoid touching your face after you touch your hair. If the oil isn't touching your skin, it can't cause the problems.

9. Watch Those Hands!

One of the easiest things you can do to avoid transferring bacteria to your face from your hands is to try not to touch your face throughout the day. Easier said than done! Without realizing it, most people typically touch their face with their hands a minimum of twenty to thirty times a day. However, it's really important to keep that type of contact to a minimum, because every time you touch your face, you layer on more dirt and bacteria that has landed on your fingers during the day from everything you touched—from the subway rail to the elevator button. And every time you do that, you could be exacerbating your challenges, no matter what skin type you have.

When you interact with other people, there's bound to be a lot of physical contact. And of course, when people care about each other, it's natural for them to want to hold hands and to touch one another. However, if you have sensitive skin or acne challenges, you'll want to keep hand-to-hand and hand-to-face contact to a minimum to avoid a skin reaction. As a compromise, if somebody is going to touch your face or your body, be sure their hands are clean. This is where your common sense should come in. Consider where the person has been and what he or she has been doing all day, and be aware that he or she might be covered in bacteria that could further harm your skin condition. I'm not telling you to live in a bubble, but it's important to remember that just because you're careful with your skin care doesn't mean everybody else is.

Also, as you may or may not know, many skin issues are tied to stress, and a lot of that stress can come from some of your interactions with other people. When you are having a stressful conversation or having a fight, you probably do things like touch your face or put your hand on your lips, and then you touch your body, your chin, and your cheeks. And as I've mentioned before, this exacerbates the transfer of bacteria that may be causing some of your skin issues. So when you're in a stressful situation at work or at home, you really need to be cognizant of how much you are touching your skin if you want to keep those challenges to a minimum.

More important, when you are stressed, the cortisol levels in your body increase and accelerate. As a result, if you have acne-prone skin, you'll have more acne. If you are in menopause, increased cortisol levels will cause a drop in your hormone levels.

If you are aging, it will actually slow down the production of collagen. So, clearly, the stress in your life can also turn up on your face. Relaxation techniques, biofeedback, and breathing training can help you cope better with life stresses and reduce their effects on your skin, making it look younger and more vibrant. As a general rule of thumb, person-to-person contact is the easiest way to transfer germs that may affect your skin, so just be conscious. And the same goes for your pets. Even though we all love to do it, try to avoid nuzzling your pet's fur. It houses a lot of harmful bacteria, as well as dirt and residue from the grass and ground, which could be wreaking havoc on your skin. So unfortunately, a close snuggle may exacerbate your situation. As an extra precaution, also be sure to wash your hands immediately after coming into contact or playing with your favorite four-legged friend. And don't let your pet on your bedding.

And last, when that all-too-common temptation to pick or pop pimples or whiteheads arises, try to resist! Touching blemishes can transfer bacteria from your fingers to your skin, potentially increasing the risk of incurring more blemishes. Improperly extracted blemishes can lead to more breakouts, infections, and even scarring. Instead, get your hands on a spot treatment designed to eliminate bacteria and soothe redness—and keep those fingers away from your magnificent mug!

10. Purse Protocol

When it comes to the purse you carry with you every day, the most important thing is to make certain it's clean and free of any bacteria that could accidentally be transferred to your skin. Think about how many times a day you reach inside your purse and how often your hands touch your face. And if the inside of your bag is full of free radicals, well, I don't have to spell out where they'll probably end up! So keeping your purse as clean as possible is actually incredibly helpful in the health of your skin.

One easy way to avoid potential harm is to take your purse to the dry cleaners and have them spot treat the inside of your bag. There is a special disinfectant a lot of them use (especially stores that are eco-friendly) that they can actually spray directly inside your purse to kill all of the invisible bacteria that's just hanging around. So whether you're using your favorite designer bag every day or use a special purse once a year, it's best to have that treatment done, because most likely, you're going to have your bags for a while and you're going to be using them all the time. So it's always good to disinfect every bag at least once a year so they're all protected and ready to use on any given occasion!

If you're going to carry makeup brushes with you, always clean them first and then place the clean brushes into a Ziploc bag that has been cleaned or into a purse that has just been cleaned. This will keep the dirt and bacteria they are exposed to down to a minimum. And when you're changing bags, you should definitely make sure the transfer from purse to purse is sanitary so you're not contaminating everything you're trying to keep clean that will actually be touching your skin at some point. Those things can cause free-radical damage and can make the acne, wrinkles, or fine lines on your face even worse.

Another thing to be conscious of is where you're placing your purse when you go to set it down when you're out and about. Every time you let it sit on public ground, such as in a restaurant, the hospital, the food court at the mall, or even the doctor's office, there are tons and tons of bacteria that will literally leech onto your bag like a barnacle on a whale. So it's always best to hang your purse on the back of your chair, put it on the couch or chair next to you, or just make certain that it doesn't touch the floor in any way. If you don't, not only is there a danger of transferring the foreign bacteria directly to your skin after you touch it, but when you place the purse that has collected the bacteria from the floor onto your car seat, your desktop, or your kitchen counter at home, those germs will then get transferred onto things that you'll most likely touch during the rest of your day, and the damaging cycle continues. So keeping your purse off the ground is the easiest and simplest way to avoid transferring any foreign bacteria from the floor onto your skin.

11. Dirty Air

If you don't properly take care of the air-filtration system in your home, the dirt, dust, and bacteria in the air may become stagnant and exacerbate or cause your skin problems. So be sure to change your house filter every ninety days for proper air filtration. Not only might poorly circulated air cause skin problems, it can also wreak havoc on your sinuses. This in turn will affect your breathing and the quality of air you are taking into your lungs. A clean filtration system, on the other hand, will make a difference in how much your body is oxygenating. And if your body is properly oxygenating, then you'll have better full-body skin!

The reason behind this is simple: the more clean air hits your skin, the more it can help your epidermis repair itself. If you're in an area with cleaner air and you're cleansing your skin multiple times and allowing it to breathe, that is going to help your skin heal and aid with the prevention of problems like wrinkles. The more oxygen that can get to your skin and into your body, the healthier it will be, and the longer the health of your cells will last.

12. Clothing Culprits

It's not uncommon for people to wear shirts, pants, or skirts several times before washing them to avoid dry-cleaning bills or doing frequent loads of laundry. However, if you have back acne or other skin challenges in places where the pre-worn clothes are touching, the dirty residue may be what's causing it. And here's why: the dirt and bacteria on your body will naturally build up each day and will transfer onto the material of the clothes you wear and get trapped in the fibers. So here's my advice: if you have serious skin problems, or very sensitive skin, you need to come to terms with the fact that the maximum number of times you can wear something to keep your body clear of acne is twice. When it comes to jeans, you might be tempted to wear them over and over to get the lived-in look and feel, but doing so can cause another set of issues. All of the oils build up around your pelvic region and get trapped in the pants, which, in turn, may create challenges, including bikini bumps, redness, rashes, and other things. Therefore, try to be mindful of how often you wear something, and you can minimize these problems.

Similar to the oxygenation theory with using a clean air filter, for aging skin, it's really important to get as much oxygen as possible to the epidermis to avoid further problems such as wrinkles and loss of elasticity in your skin. Therefore, avoid clothing made with polyesters and nylon, because those materials don't allow the skin underneath the fabric to breathe. I suggest wearing more breathable cotton fibers, because the more oxygen your epidermis gets, the more it will allow the cells to stay healthier longer, and that will ultimately give you a more youthful appearance. Plus, if you're putting an antiaging moisturizer on your skin each day, the oxygen will continue to activate the formulations in the product so it will have a better penetration effect on the skin all day long.

Creating Your New To-do List

Now that the dirty dozen of skin care has been revealed, it's time to move on to some of the positive steps you can take to further improve your skin-care routine!

Exfoliate to Radiate

Did you know that most people don't know the proper way to exfoliate, including most estheticians? When you go in for a facial, most estheticians will steam you up, cleanse your skin, and then exfoliate. But that isn't the most effective way to do it. By doing this in the reverse order after a steam (exfoliate and *then* cleanse), you'll notice an immediate difference in how clean your skin becomes.

Think about it logically: if you cleanse skin first, you're cleaning one layer and then exfoliating it away, leaving new skin that hasn't really been deeply cleaned. By exfoliating all the junk out of your skin first—the debris from the day and all the bacteria on the surface of your skin—you're actually dislodging it away, and then you are going into a second cleansing with a skin-type specific gel or cream, which is going to clean and/or treat your new skin. It shouldn't be done the other way around. Using the technique I share here is the easiest and most effective way to change up your skin-care routine, and I promise you'll see instant results!

Here is what I recommend. At home, you should have two cleansers in the shower at all times. You should have a cleanser specifically intended for exfoliation as well as another more gentle gel, foam, or cream cleanser for your specific skin type. Make sure the second product does not have an exfoliator in it (it should only be in the first product you use). You can also use a general exfoliator for the first one (not necessarily skin-care specific), so you can use whatever product is going to do the job for you and what you like for your skin. Maybe it's jojoba beads from your favorite beauty store or one of those apricot scrubs. It doesn't matter; whatever you want to use is great, and then your second cleanser will be for your skin type.

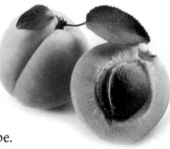

Once you've chosen your products, follow this process: exfoliate first and then cleanse. It should take you about thirty seconds to a minute for the exfoliation and thirty seconds for the cleansing. It is totally worth it; trust me! You should do this twice a day (the second time can be done with tepid water over your sink). But if you have skin that becomes sensitive or starts to break out from the extra exfoliation, you can do this process once a day. Start with doing this routine in the morning and at night and see how your skin reacts. If you find that it's too much, then cut back to once a day.

Time to Touch Up

You probably invest a good amount of time into putting yourself together and looking your best each morning. But as soon as you walk outside, with all the pollution and things in the air, your skin becomes saturated with a ton of free radicals like dirt and oil. At some point during the day, you'll probably want to touch up your makeup, but it's really important that you try to remove some of that junk from your skin first. Using an oil-blotting sheet or tissue on your face should help reduce the transfer of bacteria by lifting off the excess oil from your skin, so try to keep a pack of one or the other in your purse at all times. The most beneficial ones are the sheets infused with tea tree oil (not sheets that are powder-coated), which can help with removing some of the bacteria, in addition to removing the oil.

After dabbing your skin with an oil-blotting sheet or tissue, begin with a multipurpose product, like a multicolored powder that can be used in many ways on your face (as blush, foundation, or eye shadow) or a lipstick that can be used on your lips or as a blush substitute. Wipe it off with a tissue to remove any lingering excess dirt or bacteria and apply it as a cleansed touch-up vehicle that's going to be clean against your skin. Add or fix your color where needed and then take any product that is a skin-care mattifying liquid (such as a pore-refining product that is silicone or gel-based), put it into the palm of your hand, and mix it with a bit of antibacterial spray and then press that on top of your makeup. Doing this will actually make it look like you've taken out a brush and put more powder on to give yourself a refreshed appearance. As an added trick, you can use a dry-mist sealer (not a wet-mist sealer) to set it and make your makeup look like natural skin. You can also use this trick first thing in the morning to keep your makeup looking fresh all day.

Here's another tip for freshening up as you move from one part of your day to another. If you are running into a PTA meeting from the office or meeting someone for dinner after a long day and want to touch up your makeup, it's best to work with the same makeup you already have on rather than taking it all off and starting over. For that purpose, always keep a Ziploc baggie of tissues or cotton swabs in your purse to assist you; and as we've just discussed, if you want to carry your makeup brushes with you, be sure they are sealed inside a baggie as well to keep them clear of any bacteria floating around inside your purse.

Cotton Swabs

If you're looking for a brush substitute, cotton swabs can be a great alternative—as long as you never use them twice and are careful not to use the same swab on two different parts of your face. To get the most bang for your buck, I suggest buying the biggest type of cotton swab you can find. Using your nails, pull off the amount of cotton from whatever side of the tip you are going to be using to the point where it's going to be an effective tool for you to use. It's perfect for using once for each separate area of your face when you apply makeup.

A lot of times when I'm doing treatments on celebrities, I'll need to help them reapply their makeup after I'm done. First, I will use a sponge to apply foundation using a dabbing method to really get it into their skin. Then I will turn to my cotton swabs. I will take down the cotton so low on the first cotton swab so that I can actually do an eye-shadow lining with it; then I'll use the other side of the cotton swab for the eye shadow. I'll use a second swab and pull up the cotton and use it to 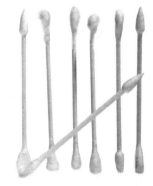 apply blush. Then I'll use a third swab for the lipstick application. It's inexpensive, quick, and most important, it's the most sanitary way to keep a person's skin flawless.

Tissue Tricks

Tissues are an excellent alternative to sponges and brushes, and can be a great application tool because they can literally help turn your hand into a brush. Each of your fingers can do a different job. Holding on to the tissue, your pinky and ring fingers are great to use all around your eye area and the smaller parts of your face for contouring, your index finger is great for blush and eyeshadow application, your middle finger is wonderful for a foundation brush for your total face, and your thumb can be used to wipe away any mistakes you make along the way. If you wrap a clean tissue around each of those fingers, you can also have a very decent and almost perfect application tool that's also going to pick up the excess debris that's left over from your cleansing and your skin-care routine. Just make sure you throw that tissue away after every use, and don't use it to blow your nose after you apply your makeup!

Ready, Set, Go!

As you can see, starting your skintervention by identifying some things in your life that might be hidden triggers for your skin issues will be monumentally useful in your journey to reinvent yourself. Not only are you helping to improve the state of your skin, but you're also creating a healthier lifestyle for your mind, body, and soul.

4

Eating Your Way
to Gorgeous

I N MY EXPERIENCE, about 90 percent of all skin issues start from within, and therefore, the way you eat affects the way you look. So now that you know your skin type and have identified a few potential exterior problem factors, let's venture into your kitchen. And whether you're more of a grab-and-go eater or a budding gourmet, it's all about what you should and shouldn't have in your pantry and refrigerator that will help keep your skin looking its best. This is not just about you buying the right things to put into your body; it's more about reconstructing the way you view food and learning how what you eat and drink can bring extra benefits and help combat those nagging skin problems. Even the tiniest changes can make the biggest difference.

Kitchen Essentials, Regardless of Skin Type

There are certain foods, liquids, and vitamins everyone needs to have on hand, regardless of your skin type. It's all about feeding your body and skin with the right nutrients to keep it functioning at maximum efficiency at all times!

Padding Your Pantry

If you're not looking at food from a low-fat or weight-management perspective, and you're just looking for solutions to skin problems, you can start by rearranging your pantry shelves according to whatever skin type you have with easy-to-grab foods that are going to make putting together face- and figure-friendly meals much more manageable. The key is having food on hand that will work with your skin to make it look the healthiest it possibly can without having to break the bank.

For all skin types, there are several items that should be in every pantry. Let's start with cooking oils. At the front of your pantry, place the most healthful oils, such as canola, olive, almond, walnut, or sesame oil. It doesn't matter if the oil is extra-virgin or not. Olive oil is one of the best choices. It's great for digestion and contains many nutrients, including vitamins A, E, and K. It's wonderful for moisturization and will give your skin that extra glow, as it actually hydrates your skin from the inside out (and yes, you can use it topically too in face masks!). If you have heavier or more fattening cooking oils or shortening, push those to the back of your pantry cabinet. Don't toss them; just use them sparingly if a recipe calls for one.

Next, I suggest filling a place on your shelf with a supply of green tea or berry-flavored tea (like raspberry, passion fruit, or any dark berry). Try to stay away from traditional black tea, because it's a diuretic and will push the water out of your system just like coffee will. The leaves of black and green tea are different —black tea contains leaves that have been completely fermented and oxidized after they've been dried, whereas green tea leaves are only steamed after they've been dried. As a result, because the black tea leaves are fermented, they contain a higher amount of caffeine (just like coffee). So while green tea does contain naturally occurring caffeine, the content is much lower and has better health benefits for your skin.

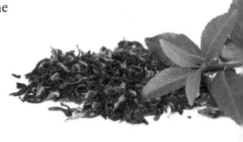

Green and berry-flavored teas contain high levels of poly-phenols, which are great anti-oxidants for overall health and body cleansing. Green tea is also great because when you drink it, it helps your body absorb the nutrients it needs and will help it release what it doesn't, keeping all of your vitamin and nutrient levels where they should be. So it's great for your body as a regulator for internal antioxidants, meaning that if your body is low in antioxidants, it actually helps to power up what you have, and if your level is too high, it will help push the excess out. It also helps your skin look and feel younger by eradicating many of those free radicals from your system. This may actually help your body break down collagen in new skin production and can help create a protective barrier internally as well.

Preserves and jams are excellent to have on hand, especially anything with berries in them, like cranberry, strawberry, or boysenberry. But be sure to read those labels and avoid brands that have excess sugars and preservatives! Preserves and jams are a great way to get the antioxidants you need because most of them are not pasteurized, and both are beneficial because they are great hydrators for the skin.

Another excellent pantry addition are pudding cups, fruit cups, or tapioca cups, which help hold more nutrients and moisture in your body because the base of each of those foods is gelatin or pectin, which are known for being moisture absorbers for the body. Some can be found in the nonrefrigerated section with things like Jell-O, but others can be found in the cold sections of your market and should be stored in your fridge.

Oatmeal is another amazing food to keep on your shelves, because it helps regulate the skin's pH balance. Oatmeal is also a natural anti-inflammatory agent, helps locks moisture into your skin, and is phenomenal for soothing your body's exterior, both when you eat it and use it topically (see Chapter 5 for an Oatmeal Skin-Polishing Scrub).

Another healthy choice is naturally processed ketchup and tomato sauces, either with whole or pureed tomatoes. These are excellent sources of lycopene, which is a great hydrator and another great antioxidant for your body. As an added bonus, they'll help give your eyes a whiter shine around the iris so you look more awake and well rested. In my opinion, when it comes to getting lycopene, just like that old saying goes with eating an apple a day, try to eat one tomato a day; it should exponentially help with hydrating and brightening your skin.

Other great items you may want to have on hand include black beans and pinto beans. All beans are great sources of fiber, which helps to regulate your system, but black beans are high in antioxidants, so reach for those first.

If you use sugar, make sure it's as minimally processed as possible. Try to get organic raw sugar if you can. But if you're trying to cut back on sugar and are trying to take care of your skin, it would be better to purchase all-natural sugar substitutes.

Last, when it comes to drinking your morning fix of caffeine, avoid instant coffee and other coffee crystals. Having a cup of coffee a day made from natural grinds is good for you in moderation. This is because caffeine helps stimulate overall circulation in your body, which is great for weight management and body firming. As mentioned earlier, caffeine is a diuretic, so drinking too much will push all the moisture out of your body. And you definitely don't want that! So be sure to find the right balance.

The Sodium Situation

If you love salt, I recommend having a small bottle of sea salt on hand. Purchase the kind that has a little bit of iodine in it versus the regular non-iodine sea salt, because you need a little bit of iodine in your system every day to synergize all the nutrients in the body to make your skin look and feel better. Use it sparingly, though. Too much sodium in your diet will give you a ticket straight to bloat city, not to mention skin issues you aren't expecting, like a puckered exterior from all that extra fluid retention!

So if you're looking for a less-salty alternative, try using spices for flavor when you can. And, of course, when you're at the grocery store, check those labels carefully for the sodium content when making purchases and stick to the low-sodium versions of the foods you buy if possible. Try to stay away from instant lunches and prepackaged noodles, because those are chock-full of salt and preservatives.

Be sure to stock your pantry with common spices that will give your food a flavorful punch while giving your skin a few added benefits. These include cumin powder, cumin seed, or cumin oil (cumin is also called black seed in some cultures). Cumin helps to fortify the renewal of fresh, healthy cells within the body, nourishes the skin from the inside out, and helps give your skin a beautiful, healthy glow by softening its texture and tone.

Next in your spice rack should be cayenne pepper, which can also be found in powder, seed, or oil form. It's great for increasing circulation, which will help detoxify your body. It helps to pull out the bad toxins, but unlike a diuretic, it doesn't wash out all the water. It's great for benefiting all skin types *except* rosacea, because it increases flushing and blushing. If you're trying to get a more youthful glow on your face, cayenne pepper helps push through any actives you have in your system, enhances clarity of the skin, and aids in generating faster cell turnover.

I also suggest having turmeric on hand. This spice has amazing anti-inflammatory properties, so it can help decrease puffiness and improve dry, sensitive skin's overall look and feel. Turmeric is a natural antiseptic and antibacterial agent, so it's also a wonderful aid when it comes to repairing damaged, broken, or scabbed skin. If you have any type of scarring or pockmarks, you can even try using it topically. It's best to use one of your moisturizers or any product that has a cream or paste base (even toothpaste!), add in a bit of turmeric, and put it directly onto your skin. Toothpaste also contains glycerin, which has great adhesion properties and will help the turmeric go right into your skin and start the healing process even faster!

Pepper of any kind (black, red, or white) is also a great spice. It not only adds flavor but also helps repair skin discoloration and hyperpigmentation. And the best part is that it doesn't

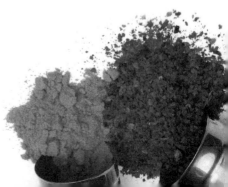

stay in your system. A lot of people don't know this, but pepper is not actually digested by the body. So you get all the benefits, including great taste, but then it flushes right out!

While not technically a spice, I also suggest that you have a supply of wheat germ on hand. Wheat germ is a great source of protein and other nutrients and has a slightly nutty flavor. You can sprinkle it on everything from your salads to chicken and even ice cream! It's a fantastic food for promoting clear and smooth skin, and for helping to increase overall collagen production and retexturizing the skin.

Juice It!

While it's not a necessary item in your skin-care regimen, a great item to have on hand is a juicer. They range in price from very costly to relatively inexpensive. Check out your local big-chain superstore for some great buys on juicers. A juicer is good for getting a dose of all of your vitamins, minerals, and other nutrients quickly and conveniently. If you're running low on time, simply toss apples, pears, and/or grapes or a combination of lettuce, celery, and tomatoes in the juicer, and drink it down. (Also, it's a good way to avoid wasting extra fruits and vegetables.)

Filling up the Fridge

Next, take a look at what you have in the fridge and move the most nutritious items to the front (and push those every-so-often treats to the back!). Fresh is best, so keep an eye on what's going to expire so you can restock it as soon as possible.

Let's begin with those incredible, edible eggs. They are good in so many different ways, but the yolk itself will help with every skin type. Because of their high sulfur content and wide array of vitamins and minerals, including a naturally occurring dose of vitamin D, eggs are great for promoting healthy hair and nails. And for the record, raw eggs are full of amazing proteins and can actually be used directly on your skin as part of your facial-care regimen! Both the yolk and white of the egg can vastly improve the appearance of tired skin on the face and under the eyes (see Chapter 5 for a do-it-yourself Firming Yolk Mask).

Believe it or not, adding a bit of mayonnaise to your diet is actually a good thing. Be sure you buy the kind made with canola oil, which is high in omega-3s and omega-6s, or even olive oil. Since mayonnaise is also made with eggs, as well as vegetable oil, it's great for your skin when eaten in moderation.

Milk is another great source of nutrients. Opt for 2 percent milk and drink one or two glasses a day. You need a little bit of the fat from the milk to synergize the actual nutrients of the liquid. Without the fat, you're only getting some of the vitamin D and other nutrients from it. The fat actually holds in a lot of the nutrients and helps your body to better absorb those vitamins right into your bloodstream. Bottom line, a little bit of fat is better than no fat.

In addition to regular milk, how about giving soymilk a whirl? I know, the word "soy" may make you cringe, but from my personal experience, I've found that chocolate, vanilla, or strawberry-flavored soymilk actually tastes better than regular milk! So I'd say that if you're a first-time soy drinker, maybe go for one of the flavored soy milks instead of the plain ones (that taste might be an acquired one!). By adding soy into your diet, you'll be able to experience some great health benefits. Certain types of isoflavonoids, like soy, are the number one ingredient that you can put into your body due to their antioxidant properties.

Also, you can get your soy from eating soy yogurt with live cultures of probiotics, or beneficial bacteria. This will help you to not only keep your digestive tract in great shape, but will also promote better texture and tone to your skin, making it more radiant. Soy will also help synergize all the other nutrients you eat and drink for the best overall skin benefits.

If you don't enjoy soy yogurt, be sure to have low-fat yogurt that contains live cultures on hand instead. The probiotics will help keep an optimum balance of good bacteria in your stomach, which helps you stay regular, detoxify, and stay healthier. The more regular you are, the better your entire system, including your skin! And the more you can push out the toxins from your body, the better your skin is going to look at any age.

If you love sour cream like me, then indulge in the full-fat version and only use a dollop here or there. The reason for this is because the fat version of sour cream has high levels of lactic acid, which is wonderful for helping to even out melanin (skin pigment), which helps with hyperpigmentation problems and helps even out skin tone. And for those ladies who are eating for two, evening out melanin can also help with the look of a "pregnancy mask"—the uneven discolored spots on the face caused by pregnancy hormones. But in general, having the lactic acid in your system will help make your skin look brighter and younger when you are exfoliating every day. Using products containing lactic acid that are applied directly to your skin will actually increase these benefits, and you'll end up with skin that really glows.

When it comes to liquids, the best ones for your skin are any type of rich, dark fruit juices (look for the concentrated or low-calorie versions), including grape, cranberry apple, or even juice from pomegranates or blueberries (or juices of the lesser known açaí berry, noni fruit, goji berry, guanabana fruit, or lychee fruit). These fruits are also considered natural humectants (a substance that promotes moisture retention) and will put extra doses of polyphenols and other antioxidants into your body. The humectant that I like to eat, drink, and use in skin-care products the most is açaí, because it naturally helps to support healthy collagen development. As the superman of antioxidants, açaí is a holistic and powerful extract that helps reduce fine lines and wrinkles, and provides skin with a beautiful, healthy glow. For many people, drinking liquids containing any of these humectants for one week makes a major difference in the reduction of dark circles and puffiness around their eyes and skin! In addition, camu camu juice is great for your skin as well.

I hope that it goes without saying that you should have plenty of water on your refrigerator shelves. Drinking tap water is fine, but water that has been purified by a home filtration system (whether via the tap or in a pitcher in the fridge) is even better. Be sure to have lots of moisture-rich fruits in the fridge like apples, cantaloupes, watermelons, and other melons, as well as strawberries and other berries, which all have high antioxidant content. In addition, stock your shelves with gelatin snacks like Jell-O. Gelatin helps with overall radiance and glow of your skin, especially for people who can't tolerate using moisturizers—like people who have combination to oily skin at an older age and can't use the more emollient topical products, or people suffering from acne-prone or sensitive skin. Gelatin is an incredible solution! If you don't eat gelatin, I also recommend products containing pectin, which you can find right next to the gelatin packets or in the canned preserves section in liquid and powder form. Pectin is just as powerful as gelatin, and it's also vegetarian!

Vegetables are a must, especially leafy greens, tomatoes, peppers (all colors), and broccoli (including broccoli rabe and broccolini). High in nutrients and fiber, vegetables are really great for any skin, hair, and nail challenge. The biotin in leafy greens and vegetables is excellent at keeping moisture in your body. Leafy greens will actually retain water more than that of normal liquids. And as we all know, water is one of the main components of having beautiful-looking skin.

Honey is another excellent food to have, as it is a natural antibiotic for your body. It helps to reduce bad bacteria in your mouth and throat and can also be used as a topical antibiotic.

And for you nut lovers, you'll be happy to know that peanut butter is on the must-have list, but you have to monitor how much of it you eat (depending on your personal calorie intake for the day—don't go overboard!). You can also try soy nut butter, almond butter, or sunflower seed butter. But make sure to read the labels and avoid getting the butters made from roasted soybeans, because roasting actually destroys a lot of the good nutrients. Try to get the ones made with raw or unroasted nuts. That's when you get the benefits of the actual nut and its oils for conditioning the skin. Be sure not to buy peanut butter or other nut butters that contain trans fat.

Too much sugar is not good for any skin type, so all things either made with or are straight sugar (in whatever form or variety) should be used in moderation.

Get Me an Açaí Berry, Stat!

By now you've most likely heard about the latest superfood to infiltrate today's market: the famous açaí berry! Experts are calling it one of the most nutritionally beneficial natural foods on Earth due to its incredible antioxidant properties. The berry itself is a small reddish purple fruit that comes from the açaí palm tree in Central and South America. And if you're wondering, it's absolutely a cousin of dark fruits like blueberries and cranberries!

Ingested as a stand-alone berry, juice, or gel capsule supplement, the açaí berry can help your body fight off free-radical attacks, which is what destroys cells, and can help combat aging, acne-prone, and sensitive skin. Its high levels of protein and dietary fiber, as well as high level of omega-6 and omega-9 fatty acids, provide many of the important and essential nutrients your body needs to be at its healthiest.

As an added bonus, the açaí berry has been proven to increase your energy, strengthen your immune system, detoxify your body, and give you healthier skin from head to toe.

Vitamin and Mineral Supplements

Now we'll take a look at which vitamins and minerals ensure an even healthier way of life, which will ultimately be reflected in your skin. For every skin type, people need to be sure that they have certain vitamins on hand to complement their diet: vitamin C, vitamin E, and vitamins B3, B6, and B12, including biotin. You also need to have sorbic acid, as well as zinc, magnesium, and calcium, not to mention that all-important açaí berry supplement. All of these can be found in nearly every multivitamin/mineral, but they will not be absorbed as well into your body if they are in a compressed form like a pill. Pills are not 100 percent bioavailable to your body, which means they won't be completely absorbed into your bloodstream. You are better off taking vitamins and minerals in gel form or as loose powder. Of course, you can also put a liquid version into your water, because this is the fastest way it's going to get the nutrients into your bloodstream. But if you want to use the pills that you already have in your cabinet, you can grind them up really well with a mortar and pestle and put them into your favorite liquid of choice. It can be anything from cranberry juice to orange juice to water, whatever you have handy. When you crush them like this, they are absorbed into your system faster because your body won't have to work as hard to break them down.

Next on the list are fish oils, which are great for increasing the overall health of your skin and conditioning your hair and nails. Fish oil can also help with free-radical reduction and smoothing out lines and wrinkles on your face. The best fish to eat are trout, herring, sardines, tilapia, mackerel, and salmon. If you don't like fish, you can buy a high-quality fish oil supplement at most grocery stores or health food stores. You can also use flaxseed, which is widely available in drugstores and vitamin shops. It contains all the omega-3s, 6s, and 9s found in fish oil, plus a barrage of other oils that are excellent for all skin types. While fish oil and flaxseed oil are not identical, they do have similar benefits. But taking both every day is actually the best way to go.

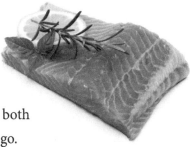

Food Cures for Specific Conditions

In addition to the main staples everyone should have in their kitchen to promote healthy skin, there are also a few additional items to consider that can help with more specific skin problems. Let's take a look at them.

Battling Aging Skin and Boosting Your Outer Radiance

In your skintervention against aging skin, one of the best foods to snack on is nuts, such as almonds, pumpkin seeds, sunflower seeds, and Brazil nuts. Almonds, in particular, reap a tremendous amount of health benefits, including preventing the premature appearance of wrinkles, blackheads, pimples, and dry skin, and will even help get rid of those dark circles under your eyes. Both pumpkin and sunflower seeds are great sources of fiber and vitamin E, which are excellent antioxidants that help diminish the appearance of stretch marks and the redness associated with erythema and rosacea. And Brazil nuts, also high in vitamins A and E, can help prevent skin dryness, which contributes to antiaging. They also contain the mineral selenium, which will improve the elasticity of your skin and help fight off skin infections. Other staples for this skin condition include grape seed extract and the spices curry and saffron, which will help alleviate dry skin and inflammation within your body and are excellent sources for flavor when you cook.

And as mentioned, green tea is great for increasing collagen production in the body, and it contains vitamin C, so it's great for antiaging. And don't forget preserves made with gelatin and pectin, which increase the elasticity in your skin and help firm up your exterior.

For a woman who wants to look younger and get back that youthful glow, eating leafy green vegetables is the way to go. The best choices are spinach, radicchio, Swiss chard, romaine, butter leaf, arugula, bok choy, collard greens, and iceberg (if you can't find any of the others). You will gain the biggest benefits if you eat these lettuce leaves uncooked, but do make sure they are thoroughly washed and cleaned.

For fine lines and wrinkles, eat foods with high levels of malic acid, which is closely related to citric acid, a form of vitamin C. Malic acid can be found in a variety of fruits and berries, including cherries, tomatoes, blackberries, blueberries, boysenberries, red grapes, goji berries, and black currant, but especially in apples. Citric acid in citrus fruit, such as lemons, limes, and oranges, can also be applied to your skin to help reduce the appearance of liver spots on the face (see Chapter 5's When Life Gives You Lemons for using lemons in home treatments).

In addition to all of the foods mentioned, one of the key items you'll want to purchase is an açaí berry supplement, either in a chewable tablet or gelcap. With all of its beneficial nutrients, this berry is believed to actually help slow down the aging process! And who doesn't want that?

Ditching Your Dry or Sensitive Skin

If your skin is dry, cracked, or sensitive, you want to make certain that you give your body higher levels of vitamin C. Vitamin

C externally (through a gelcap) and internally helps close your pores, and by doing that, it will actually help you mitigate the capillaries in your skin and will help suppress those little red lines that pop up on your nose and cheeks.

If you have enlarged pores, avoid dilators in your skin, such as excess niacin. Instead, try to get your antioxidants and vitamins from foods, like raspberries, strawberries, açaí, and goji, as well as flaxseed and sesame seeds.

If your skin is dry, your cells need to be hydrated. Lock in as much moisture as possible by drinking lots of liquids. But don't forget about adding fruit cups to your diet, which are a portable and tasty way to hold in some of that much-needed moisture for your skin. Milk, with its lactic acid content, is also fantastic to both drink and use externally (yes, you can wash your face with it too! See Chapter 5). Milk is an amazing exfoliant and cleanser for your skin, and when you drink it, the fat and proteins it contains will provide your skin with a softer, suppler feeling.

Make sure you consume a lot of citrus fruits in your diet, as well as plenty of yellow and orange vegetables. These contain high levels of the antioxidant beta-carotene, which your body will convert to vitamin A. To keep your skin looking smooth and healthy, try eating foods rich in sulfur, such as garlic, onion, eggs, and asparagus.

You also want to have a lot of biotin in your system, which is great for keratin production and growth of your skin, nails, and hair, and will give you shine and strength and that much-sought-after glossy finish. But because it's not found in many foods, you should supplement your diet with a gel capsule of biotin. While biotin can be found in a B complex vitamin, you won't be getting the right amount of actual biotin complex needed to help with sensitive skin, so adding a supplement is your best bet.

Abolishing Acne or Oily Skin

To help reduce skin problems associated with rosacea and acne, you want to make sure that your skin is infused with isoflavonoids and polyphenols, which come from lots of berries, especially anything from the red berry family, such as pomegranates and grape seeds. These will help pull out all the toxins in your body and help clarify and control oil on the skin.

You'll also want a lot of vitamin E in your body, which you can get from foods like nuts and broccoli, as well as in a pill or a gelcap form. This will be a huge help when it comes to the clarity of your skin.

Eating foods with anti-inflammatory agents in them is also important. Soy products, ginger, mushrooms, and goji berries will work to reduce inflammation in your skin. Walnuts, flaxseed, and olive oil all contain rich amounts of omega-3 oils, which are also powerful anti-inflammatory agents.

Believe it or not, dark chocolate is actually very good for skin with acne because of its high antioxidant content. In addition, try to include other anti-inflammatory foods in your diet, like pomegranate and goji berries, as well as a well-balanced mix of vitamins A, B, C, D, E, and zinc.

When grocery shopping, look for foods that are high in vitamin A, such as spinach, collard greens, or any green leafy vegetables, which are good hydrators and detoxifiers. (Too much vitamin A can be harmful, so speak with your doctor about the correct amounts for you.) Eating foods like pomegranates or dark berries will help keep your skin hydrated in the right way.

If oily skin is an issue, limit the amount of hydrogenated oil (such as vegetable oil or margarine) you are using to cook with because it will ultimately end up in your body. While healthy monounsaturated oils are great for your health, try to maintain a normal to average level versus an excessive amount. For example, cook with oil every other day instead of every day. Baking or steaming your foods is a fantastic alternative to cooking with oil.

Firming the Flab

If you've recently lost weight or given birth, you may have some skin that needs firming. For this condition, you want to find foods that contain more fatty acids, which help with skin's elasticity, such as avocados, fish, and nuts (like almonds, Brazil nuts, cashews, and pecans). Some other skin-firming foods are ones that are packed with vitamins and minerals, especially vitamin K, such as kale, spinach, beets, turnips, mustard greens, Brussels sprouts, and onions, as well as grape seed, which is wonderful for overall collagen stimulation. Hyaluronic acid is also very important, and you can find it in foods such as green peppers, Brussels sprouts, broccoli, oranges, potatoes, and soy. You can also buy concentrated versions of hyaluronic acid in both pill and liquid forms at your local vitamin shop as well as in your topical products. The enzymes found in both papaya and guava are wonderful for helping to stimulate the firming memory of the skin. You can eat them both dry and fresh. As an added bonus, the enzymes in papaya and guava will help reduce the appearance of stretch marks. Vitamin E is also very good for stretch marks, so eat vitamin E–rich foods, such as almonds, wheat germ, sunflower seeds, turnip greens, tomatoes, and avocados, and supplement your skin care with a gel tab as well. If you're currently pregnant, please consult your doctor before taking any supplements. Instead, you can try using a topical cream containing vitamin E to help you receive those benefits.

Always carry a bottle of water to keep your body hydrated. If you want to make your water even more healthful, heat up some green tea and then cool it down; once it's cool, add it to your water bottle. The warmth of the water will increase your circulation and help all the antioxidants, vitamins, and minerals you've ingested be better absorbed. Green tea contains anthocyanins and polyphenols, which help with detoxification. It's also wonderful for weight management because it actually helps your internal cell walls hold onto that moisture content.

Last, including a niacinamide pill (which is a form of vitamin B) and high levels of grape seed extract in your daily routine can help with the firming memory of the body to maintain its silhouette if you have one, and it's a great way to help you get one if you don't already! And just a side note, niacin itself does cause flushing, so this pill could have the same effect on your skin, but it's nothing to worry about.

Doing all of the things I've just mentioned will work together to help your body become tauter and keep it regulated as you continue to lose weight or try to maintain your new physique.

Managing Menopausal Skin

You may suddenly find yourself having acne breakouts in your forties or fifties or witness your skin doing things it has never done before, which can all be attributed to the onset of menopause. So to help with this particular situation, try the suggestions listed previously in both the antiaging and acne categories. Combining the foods in both sections will help immensely!

But if you want just one or two things to try because you're getting hormonal breakouts as you age, try adding hormone regulators into your diet. Hormone regulators include soy (which contains isoflavonoids) and black cohosh, which you can get in a gel or capsule form. Hormone regulators help keep your hormone levels balanced. And last, the nutrients you need to alleviate menopausal symptoms are actually a bit different from nutrients that can help with premenstrual symptoms. Menopause is a big life transition. To help your skin glow throughout this transition, ask your esthetician or nutritionist how adding the following supplements to your diet can help you: black cohosh, dong quai, isoflavonoids and other phytoestrogens, red clover, licorice, iron, and evening primrose oil.

PMS SOS

No one likes to talk about PMS. Maybe that's why so many women suffer in secrecy with their symptoms every month. Yet as women know all too well, symptoms aren't easily hidden; in fact, they often show up all over the face. Complexion imperfections, blotchiness, fatigue, and skin tone unevenness are just some of the challenges associated with "PMS skin." From hormonal breakouts to a complexion that is in constant flux for days on end, your rebelling skin may need an extra dose of TLC just before your monthly cycle begins.

If you're looking for products that can help when signs of PMS erupt on your skin, try the BORBA PMS Skin Rescue System, as well as the BORBA PMS Rescue Beverage Crystals, to rejuvenate, retexturize, retighten, and renourish facial skin. In addition, foods rich in the following nutrients will help: calcium, folate, iodine, magnesium, niacin, riboflavin, thiamin, vitamin B6, vitamin B12, vitamin D, vitamin E, and zinc.

Skin-Savvy Recipes

Now that you know the advantages of certain foods, I want to give you some ideas about how to cook with many of the ingredients we've talked about in previous chapters. I'm about to share with you several of my favorite recipes that include some of the best and most beneficial ingredients to use in cooking and what you can use as substitutions to make the dishes work for your skin-care needs.

We all have good days and bad days, so these are just a few suggestions of things you can incorporate into your diet to enhance your health. I'm not trying to tell you to change your diet completely but just to be open to exploring some new foods.

I know you're going to eat bread and have an occasional dessert. This is a way for you to continue to do that, but in a better way. Most of us love ice cream, and that's why I've included one of my recipes for a healthy alternative. Most people love fried foods, and that's why I've included one of my spring roll recipes. If you're going to treat yourself to these things, why not reap a few health benefits at the same time? Almost any food can be somewhat healthy if you prepare it properly or swap in a few skin-friendly ingredients. By creating some of these yummy recipes, you won't have to feel any sort of guilt as you sip and nibble your way to beautiful skin.

Borba-Cado Spring Rolls

Function: This will be a hit at your next party. From the vitamins, amino acids, the omega-3 and omega-6 in the avocados, and the lycopene in the tomatoes, this is chock-full of healthy ingredients. It's a great appetizer that won't contribute to a breakout.

INGREDIENTS:

2 ripe avocados

juice of 1 lime

3 tablespoons chopped sundried tomatoes

3 tablespoons finely chopped onion

2 tablespoons finely chopped cilantro

$^1/_2$ cherimoya (skinned and seeded) (or 1 packet Replenishing Lychee Fruit Antioxidant Crystalline Drink Mix)

1 teaspoon Thai Massaman curry paste

6 egg roll wrappers

7 ounces peanut oil

SAUCE:

2 tablespoons dry white wine

$1^1/_2$ tablespoons Thai Massaman curry paste

2 tablespoons peanut oil

1 Mash avocados with lime juice in a medium mixing bowl just until chunky. Then add the tomatoes, red onion, cilantro, cherimoya, and curry paste until combined.

2 Lay one egg roll wrapper on a cutting board and along the long side of the egg roll wrapper.

3 Place 2 tablespoons of the mixture ½ inch from the edge. Fold in the two shorter ends and then fold over the ½-inch border over the avocado mixture and roll until the wrapper is enclosing the avocado mixture completely and it is in a log shape. Lay seam side down and continue doing this with the other five wrappers. These can be made up to four hours in advance and kept at room temperature.

4 To serve, heat the peanut oil in a medium frying pan until very hot and the egg rolls sizzle when added. Add two rolls at a time, frying 2 to 3 minutes per side until the wrapper is browned and crisped. Remove, drain on paper towels, and cut in half on the diagonal into two or three pieces to serve.

5 To make the sauce, boil the wine for three minutes until slightly reduced and then mix in the Thai paste and oil. Serve alongside the spring rolls.

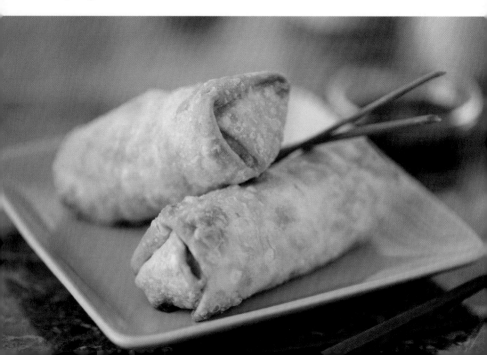

Borba-que

Function: A simple recipe that gives head-to-toe skin benefits, especially from the high protein content, vitamin E and C, and the antioxidants. This dish is especially great for aging skin.

INGREDIENTS:

20 large shrimp

1 cup olive oil

juice of 3 lemons

¼ cup soy sauce

¼ cup finely chopped parsley

¼ cup lychee syrup with pulp solids (or 1 packet of Replenishing Lychee Fruit Antioxidant Crystalline Drink Mix)

3 tablespoons fresh tarragon, chopped

1 With sharp scissors, cut down the back of each shrimp shell and remove the black vein, keeping the shell on and intact. Wash the shrimp thoroughly and place them in a large bowl.

2 Pour the olive oil, lemon juice, soy sauce, parsley, lychee syrup, and tarragon over the shrimp. Let the shrimp stand for two hours, tossing occasionally to marinate equally.

3 Arrange the shrimp in basket grills, or thread through skewers, and cook over hot coals for five to six minutes, turning twice. The shrimp should be tender and moist with lightly charred shells.

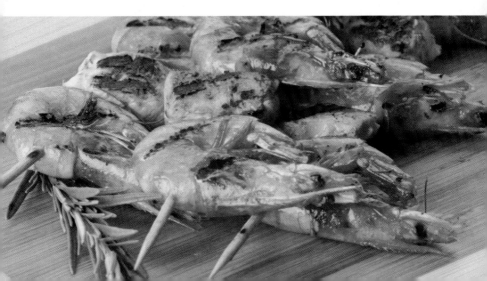

"Skin"ful Nachos

Function: I love snacking. I made this recipe for a fun snack that's easy to make. People with oily skin love this recipe because it's the one nacho recipe that doesn't make their skin feel greasy when they're done eating it!

INGREDIENTS:

6 wheat tortillas (rich in selenium)

1 tablespoon of canola oil (rich in fatty acids)

$\frac{1}{2}$ cup shredded low-fat cheddar cheese (rich in vitamins A and D and calcium)

6 diced black olives (rich in monounsaturated fat and vitamin E)

$\frac{1}{2}$ tablespoon flaxseed powder

1 tablespoon sour cream

Preheat the oven to 350 degrees Fahrenheit.

1 Cut each tortilla into eight pieces and place them on a baking sheet. Drizzle them with the canola oil and bake for 10 minutes.

2 When the chips start to get crisp, sprinkle on the cheddar cheese and black olives and put them back in the oven just long enough for the cheese to melt.

3 For the topping, mix the flaxseed powder with the sour cream and serve.

Borba Skin-Balancing Strips

Function: This delicious dish is rich in antioxidants and vitamins A, C, and E, which are great for all skin types, especially aging skin.

INGREDIENTS:

2 mangoes, peeled, seeded, and chopped

3 tablespoons honey

$\frac{1}{4}$ cup lime juice

$\frac{1}{4}$ cup olive oil

3 tablespoons soy sauce

$\frac{1}{2}$ cup fresh pomegranate juice (or $\frac{1}{2}$ cup water mixed with Clarifying Pomegranate Antioxidant Crystalline Drink Mix)

6 boneless, skinless chicken breasts, halved

1   Place the mangoes, honey, and lime juice into a blender; cover and blend until smooth. Place the mango mixture in a covered bowl in the refrigerator.

2   Mix the oil, soy sauce, and pomegranate juice into a small bowl to make a marinade.

3   Cut the chicken into strips. Pour the marinade over the chicken in a glass pan. Cover and marinate for four hours.

4   Set the oven to broil. Thread the chicken onto metal skewers and cook 8 to 10 minutes, turning once, until done. Serve with the mango sauce.

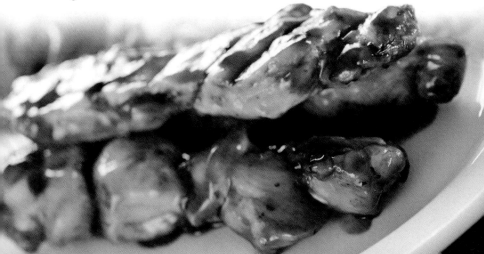

Pomegranate Chicken

Function: This is my number one favorite recipe for attaining clarity and alleviating breakout challenges. The high amount of antioxidants and antimicrobial ingredients make this dish your best bet for when clear skin is absolutely necessary.

INGREDIENTS:

2 cups pomegranate juice

2 cups chicken stock

2 tablespoons honey

1¹/₂ cloves of garlic

Kosher salt, to taste

pepper, to taste

truffle oil (or olive oil if you
   don't have truffle)

4 stalks minced green onion

1 whole chicken (3–5 lbs.)

1 In a saucepan, add the pomegranate juice, chicken stock, honey, and the garlic, and reduce the mixture to a glaze at medium heat for about an hour. Season with salt and pepper when the glaze has reduced.

2 Apply the truffle oil liberally to the outside of a medium-sized whole chicken. Season the outside and inside with kosher salt and black pepper. Rub the outside of the chicken with four blades of the minced green onion, then baste the outside of the chicken with the pomegranate glaze.

3 Cook in the oven at 450 degrees for one hour, then reduce the heat to 350 degrees and continue cooking for another 30 minutes. Remove from the oven and let cool for 10 to 15 minutes before serving.

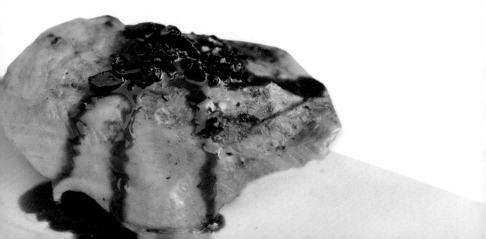

High-Energy Salmon Steak

Function: The high amount of protein and omegas in this dish make it one of my favorites for quickly fixing dry or sallow-looking skin.

INGREDIENTS:

6 ounces salmon steak (high in protein, fatty acids, and vitamins B and E)

4 crushed peppercorns

1 ounce extra-virgin olive oil

juice of 1 lemon, separated into two portions

¹⁄₄ teaspoon turmeric

SAUCE:

2 baby carrots

1 vitamin E capsule (approximately 400–1,000 IU)

1 vitamin B capsule (approximately 2,000 IU)

Sprig of parsley

Zest of lemon

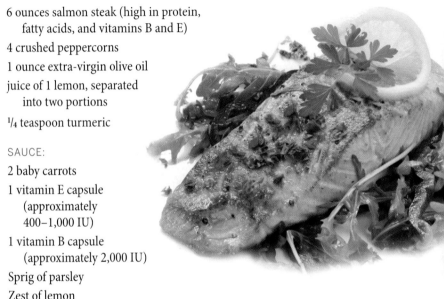

1 Coat one side of the salmon steak with 4 crushed peppercorns and the olive oil, and then splash on half of the lemon juice mixed with ¹⁄₄ teaspoon of turmeric.

2 Bake for 20 minutes at 300 degrees and let it sit for a few minutes while you prepare the sauce.

3 For the sauce, blend the 2 baby carrots, the remaining lemon juice, and the liquid from the vitamin E and vitamin B capsules. (Don't worry, the bitter taste will be a complement to the fiery black pepper and tangy lemon juice.)

4 To serve, pour over the salmon steak and garnish with a sprig of parsley and the zest of the lemon.

Chocolate-Covered Borberries

Function: This treat may taste sinful, but the high levels of antioxidants and vitamins will add life back into aging skin.

INGREDIENTS:

Liquid from 2 vitamin E capsules—approximately 2,000 IU
(or 1 packet of Firming Guanabana Fruit Antioxidant
Crystalline Drink Mix)

2 pints strawberries

1 cup semisweet dark chocolate chips

1 Line a large baking sheet with waxed paper.

2 Rinse the strawberries and pat dry.

3 Combine the vitamin E liquid with the chocolate chips and melt as package directs.

4 Holding the strawberry by the stem, dip it into the chocolate to cover about ³/₄ of the berry. Lay the strawberry on a baking sheet. Repeat with remaining strawberries.

5 Refrigerate the berries until the chocolate is set.

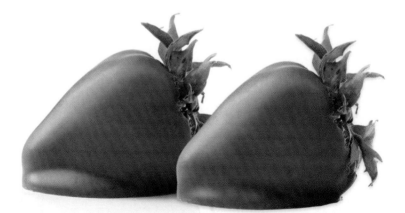

Borba Frigid

Function: *This is a festive and fun recipe that hydrates your skin. Try making this after a long, hot summer day for a cool skin replenishment.*

INGREDIENTS:

8 cups chopped, seeded watermelon

$^1/_2$ cup lychee juice, either straight from the berry or from a can (or 2 packets of Replenishing Lychee Fruit Antioxidant Crystalline Drink Mix)

$1^1/_2$ tablespoons lime juice

1 cup light honey

$^1/_2$ teaspoon ground cardamom

$^1/_2$ package unflavored gelatin

$^1/_2$ cup nonfat plain yogurt

12 mint leaves

1 Place the watermelon, lychee, and lime juice in a blender and puree.

2 Set a colander over a large bowl and pour the pureed watermelon through it, separating the juice from the pulp.

3 Place the watermelon juice, honey, cardamom, and gelatin in a large saucepan over medium-high heat and reduce it down until you get a decent syrup. Let cool.

4 Pour the watermelon mixture into a shallow pan or ice-cube tray and freeze until it resembles slush (about $1^1/_4$ hours).

5 Whisk the yogurt into the watermelon slush and then return it to the freezer. Allow the mixture to freeze solid (about two hours), stirring every half hour to break up ice crystals.

6 To serve, cut the sherbet into large chunks and puree very briefly in a blender or food processor. Spoon into dessert glasses, garnish with a mint leaf, and serve.

Borbanana Bread

Function: I love taking a classic like banana bread and adding my own skin-healthy twist. With my recipe additions, you won't taste the difference, but you'll see it on your skin. The flaxseed powder and bananas will both help your skin look smoother and will help reduce inflammation.

INGREDIENTS:

5 tablespoons butter

6 vitamin E capsules—approximately 2,000–4,000 IU for full loaf, squeezed and casing discarded (or 2 packets of Replenishing Lychee Fruit Antioxidant Crystalline Drink Mix)

$^1/_2$ cup granulated sugar

$^1/_2$ cup firmly packed light brown sugar

1 large egg

2 egg whites

1 teaspoon vanilla extract

$1^1/_2$ cups mashed ripe bananas

$1^1/_2$ cups of all-purpose flour

$^1/_2$ cup flaxseed powder

1 teaspoon baking soda

$^1/_2$ teaspoon salt

$^1/_4$ teaspoon baking powder

$^1/_2$ cup heavy cream

1 cup chopped walnuts

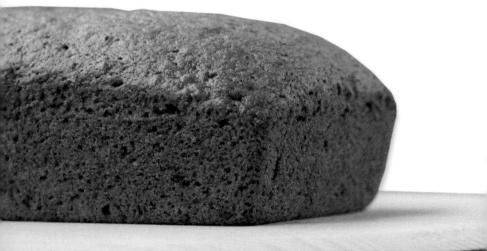

1 Preheat oven to 350 Fahrenheit. Spray the bottom only of a 9 × 5 × 3–inch loaf pan with nonstick cooking spray.

2 Beat the butter in large bowl with an electric mixer at medium speed and add the liquid from the vitamin E capsules. Add the granulated sugar and brown sugar and beat well until mixed.

3 Add the egg, egg whites, and vanilla and beat until well blended. Add the mashed banana and beat on high speed for 30 seconds.

4 Combine the flour, flaxseed powder, baking soda, salt, and baking powder in a medium bowl.

5 Add the flour mixture to the butter mixture alternately with cream, ending with flour mixture.

6 Add the walnuts to the batter and mix well.

7 Pour the batter evenly into the prepared loaf pan. Bake until browned (about 1 hour 15 minutes). Insert a toothpick near the center and make sure it comes out clean.

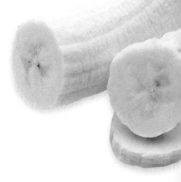

Borbonade

Function: If you are going to drink, which dries the skin, adding the pomegranate juice or my Skin Balance Water will help to strengthen your immune system, remove toxins, and improve clarity of the epidermis.

INGREDIENTS:

1.5 ounces vodka

4.5 ounces lemonade

.75 ounce pomegranate juice (or .75 ounce Clarifying Pomegranate Skin Balance Water)

1 lemon slice

Pour all of the ingredients into a tall glass filled with ice. Stir and garnish with a lemon wheel.

The Sponge

Function: Lychee fruit is known for boosting moisture levels, which keeps your skin smooth and firm.

INGREDIENTS:

1.8 ounces of vodka

1.8 ounces lychee syrup with pulp (or 1.8 ounces of Replenishing Lychee Fruit Skin Balance Water)

1 lemon

Fill a cocktail shaker halfway with ice. Combine all ingredients and shake well. Strain the mixture into a chilled, stemmed cocktail glass and garnish with a lemon twist.

Fountain of Youth

Function: Grapes and açaí berries help soften fine lines and wrinkles, increase elasticity, and renew skin's natural glow.

INGREDIENTS:

1.8 ounces of vodka

1.8 ounces of dark grape juice concentrate (or 1.8 ounces of Age Defying Açaí Berry Skin Balance Water)

Fill a cocktail shaker halfway with ice. Combine all ingredients and shake well. Strain the mixture into a chilled, stemmed cocktail glass and garnish with a lemon twist.

Flawless

Function: Pomegranate is helpful in removing toxins and improving clarity of the epidermis.

INGREDIENTS:

1.8 ounces of vodka

1.8 ounces of fresh-pressed pomegranate seeds (or 1.8 ounces of Clarifying Pomegranate Skin Balance Water)

Fill a cocktail shaker halfway with ice. Combine all ingredients and shake well. Strain the mixture into a chilled, stemmed cocktail glass and garnish with a lemon twist.

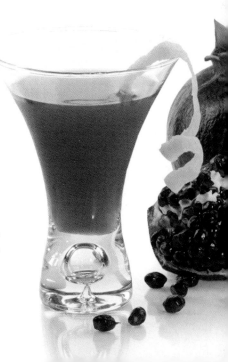

The Concealer

Function: Lychee fruit and tomatoes help reduce the appearance of redness and irritated skin.

INGREDIENTS:

1.8 ounces of vodka

1.8 ounces of tomato puree (or 1.8 ounces of Replenishing Lychee Fruit Skin Balance Water)

Fill a cocktail shaker halfway with ice. Combine all ingredients and shake well. Strain the mixture into a chilled, stemmed cocktail glass, add a dash of pepper sauce, and garnish with a lemon twist.

Wonder Twins

Function: Both blueberries and açaí berries soften fine lines and wrinkles, purge impurities, and improve skin clarity and radiance.

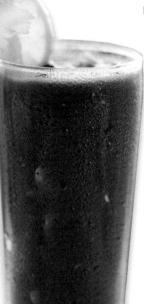

INGREDIENTS:

1.8 ounces of vodka

1.8 ounces of fresh-pressed blueberry juice with pulp (or 1.8 ounces of Clarifying Pomegranate Skin Balance Water or Age Defying Açaí Berry Skin Balance Water)

Fill a cocktail shaker halfway with ice. Combine all ingredients and shake well. Strain the mixture into a chilled, stemmed cocktail glass and garnish with a lemon twist.

Pomevation

Function: Pomegranates are excellent in removing toxins and improving clarity of the epidermis.

INGREDIENTS:

1.8 ounces of vodka

6 ounces of tonic

.75 ounce pomegranate juice from concentrate (or .75 ounce of Clarifying Pomegranate Skin Balance Water)

Fill a highball glass with ice; add the vodka and pomegranate juice and garnish with a twist of lime.

Borba Skin-gestible

Function: Blueberries and açaí berries are a powerful combination that helps soften fine lines and wrinkles, increases elasticity, and renews your skin's natural glow.

INGREDIENTS:

1 cup frozen organic strawberries

1 cup orange juice

1 cup blueberries (or 1 cup Age Defying Açaí Berry Skin Balance Water)

1 teaspoon fresh lemon juice

1 cup light rum

Combine all ingredients in a blender and puree until smooth. Serve with a garnish of fresh fruit.

Complexion-Enhancing
Chocolate Milk

. . . .

Function: This drink is a
delicious source of vitamins
and is a guilt-free treat when
you're craving chocolate.

INGREDIENTS:

1 ounce dark chocolate

7 ounces 2% milk

1 ounce vanilla almond milk

Heat the dark chocolate
in a microwave-safe bowl
in the microwave for about
8 seconds. Pour the heated
chocolate into the milk
and then add the vanilla
almond milk. Stir until the
chocolate is incorporated
fully into the milk and
enjoy.

5

Pamper Yourself Beautiful: Do-It-Yourself Facials, Spas, and Treatments

NOW THAT I'VE GIVEN YOU some helpful hints for specific topical issues, it's time to dive into things you can do to help keep yourself looking great, both at home and on the go!

If you can't get to a glorious and relaxing spa, or if you just don't want to spend hundreds of dollars, here are a few easy tricks you can use to improve your skin at home without the expensive price tag.

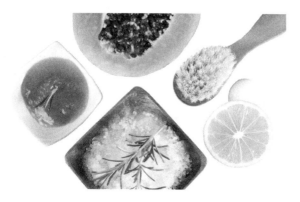

DIY Pore-Opening Scrub

1/2 teaspoon baking soda

1/4 tablespoon raw brown sugar (or white sugar)

Mix the baking soda with the sugar and then rub it onto your face. Leave it on until your skin starts to tingle, which can be anywhere from 30 seconds to 5 minutes. Wash the mixture off with warm water. The sugar scrub will open up your pores, and the baking soda will not only help clear up skin imperfections, but will help mattify your skin as well.

Oatmeal Skin-Polishing Scrub

3/4 cup dry oatmeal

1/2 cup honey

Mix the oatmeal with the honey until it's well blended. Rub the mixture onto your face or body for a few minutes and then rinse off in the shower. Your skin will glow and your wallet will shine!

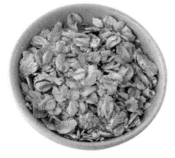

Alleluia Paraffin Mitts

Nickel-sized amount of Vaseline, olive oil, or shea butter

Pre-cling plastic wrap

This is a great way to fix dry skin. Simply apply the Vaseline, olive oil, or shea butter to the area you want to treat, for example, your hands or feet. Cover each treated area with precut cling wrap. Finally, cover your hands or feet with clean, dry socks to lock in deep moisture and suppleness overnight.

Vita-Vegi Antiaging Mask

1 large avocado (contains antiaging omegas)

1 vitamin E soft gel (approximately 400 IU)

Dash cayenne pepper (for thermal stimulation)

1 tablespoon honey (for antimicrobial effect)

In a bowl, mash together the avocado, the gel from the vitamin E, the cayenne pepper, and 1 tablespoon of honey. Once the ingredients are completely mixed, apply a thick coat to your face and neck area and leave on for about thirty minutes. Wash the mixture off with a damp washcloth, and your skin will feel smooth and tight. Repeat once a week.

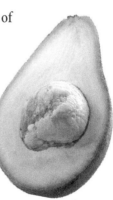

Clarifying Chocolate Mask

3/4 cup lukewarm water

1 tablespoon honey

1 tablespoon chocolate syrup

1 cup instant oatmeal

Stir all of the ingredients until well blended. Apply the mixture to your face with a clean, flat paintbrush, sponge, or spoon, and let it dry for about fifteen minutes. Lightly scrub the mixture off with lukewarm water. The oatmeal will soak up excess oils and exfoliate when scrubbed away, the honey will refine your pores while killing surface bacteria, and the chocolate polyphenols help with fine lines and wrinkles while soothing your senses.

Firming Yolk Mask

1 egg

1 teaspoon baking soda

Beat the egg (use the whole egg because the omegas are in the yolk) and add a teaspoon of baking soda. Brush the mixture on your face with a clean, flat brush, sponge, or spoon. Let the mixture dry for about 8 minutes and then gently wash it off with warm water. Egg yolks are high in skin-nourishing vitamins A, D, and E, as well as skin-firming protein. Baking soda is good for tightening skin and killing bacteria. Use this mask no more than twice a week.

No Wiggle Antiaging Gelatin Serum

1 tablespoon unflavored, powdered gelatin

1 tablespoon water

1 or 2 drops of olive oil

Scoop out a tablespoon of the powdered gelatin and mix it with the water and olive oil, which will create a paste. Emulsify a pearl-sized amount of the mixture in your palms and gently press into your face and neck. Use this in addition to, or in place of, your current antiaging serum or at night as an intensive weekly antiaging serum. The gelatin is made of collagen, which is the protein that gives skin elasticity, and the olive oil is ultramoisturizing.

Pretty 'N Pink Tightening Mask

1 tablespoon of Pepto-Bismol

While Pepto-Bismol is normally used to settle and soothe the stomach, you can also use it on your skin straight from the bottle as a clarifying mask. It contains salicylic acid, an ingredient that can slough off dead skin cells, work as an antiaging active, and dry up your acne. So if you're short on cash and need a quick fix for most skin issues, turn to the pink bottle and give it a whirl. Leave it on for about five minutes, but if your face starts to really tingle before then, take it off. Remove with either cold or tepid water.

DIY Facial

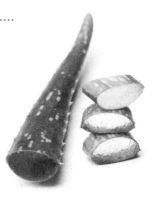

Basic Facial:

Towel

Vaporizer or pot of boiling water

1/4 cup plain Greek yogurt

1/4 cup buttermilk

For Puffy or Tired Eyes:

2 coffee filters

Freshly brewed coffee grounds

For the Ultimate Facial:

5 vitamin E capsules (approximately 1,000–2,000 IU)

Dime-sized dollop of aloe vera gel or honey

An at-home deep facial moisture wrap is as easy as looking in your pantry. This self-pampering treatment will gently exfoliate your epidermis and dissolve visible debris like blackheads and whiteheads while intensely moisturizing and providing a natural glow on your face.

Start by wrapping a towel around your face (covering it up) and carefully and safely lean over a vaporizer or pot of boiling water for three minutes to hold in the steam. This will open up the pores just like at a traditional spa and soften the debris in your skin so it can easily be massaged out. Then rinse your face with tepid water. Your next step is to mix the yogurt and buttermilk together and to apply or massage the mixture into your face. Both yogurt and buttermilk contain high concentrations of lactic acid, which is a gentle yet effective natural ingredient to smooth out the skin. Allow the mixture to remain on your skin for ten to fifteen minutes before rinsing off with warm water.

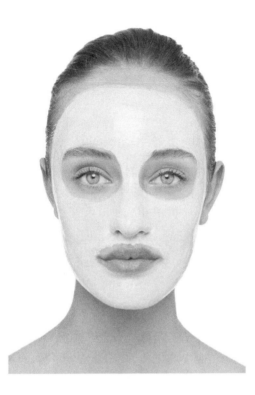

Now for your eyes: To help perk up those tired peepers, place two new coffee filter cups filled with freshly brewed coffee grounds onto your eyes for a few minutes. This will help de-puff the entire eye area so you'll look well rested. Then gently rinse your face with tepid water.

To finish out the facial and power-hydrate the skin, break open five liquid gel vitamin E capsules and combine them with the dime-sized dollop of pure aloe vera gel or honey. Massage the mixture gently into your skin and poof! A professional DIY facial in your own home! If you want extra hydration, finish off your treatment by using a pearl-sized amount of your favorite day or night moisturizer on your freshly cleansed skin.

When Life Gives You Lemons

1/2 cup sea salt

3 tablespoons honey

1 teaspoon finely grated lemon zest

This is a great treatment to brighten dull winter skin. Lemon zest combined with sea salt can bring a healthy glow to otherwise lackluster dry skin. In a medium bowl, combine the sea salt with the honey and the lemon zest until well mixed. Rub the mixture vigorously over any dry areas of your skin. The vitamin C in this mixture actually rivals any professional lactic acid treatment in a spa! It will also help to even out skin tone and minimize enlarged pores and blotchiness, so your makeup will look more natural. You can do this treatment every other day.

Here's another way to use lemons on your skin as a healthy alternative to a pricey salon experience. Start by rolling four room-temperature lemons back and forth for a minute or two. Then cut the lemons in half and squeeze the juice and the pulp into a bowl or measuring cup. Mix in one foil packet of liquid pectin, which you can find at any grocery store in the gelatin aisle. Apply the mixture liberally to your entire face, neck, décolleté, and back of your hands. When your skin starts to tingle, that's your cue to wash the mixture off (but do not leave it on your skin for more than five minutes). The pectin will plump up the skin and smooth out your skin texture, while the lemons will brighten skin, increase radiance, and even out skin tone. Glowing skin guaranteed! You can do this every day if desired.

Going Bananas
....

1 banana

Vaseline, chilled overnight in the refrigerator

The next time you make a banana smoothie or eat a banana, don't throw away the peel. You can give your tired eyes the slip with this simple recipe. Take a banana out of the peel and run a large spoon from the top to the bottom of the peel until you strip it of its internal fibers, which are those white strips that can be found between the banana and the inside of the peel itself. Mix the husk and peel with a quarter-sized amount of cold Vaseline. Apply the mixture to your eyelids and on the top of your eyebrows. Allow it to set for five minutes and then gently wipe it off with a tissue. You will be astounded by the reduction of the loose skin and the wide-awake look you will achieve from doing something so simple! Make sure that you have removed the excess Vaseline from your eyes prior to any makeup application; you can use a makeup-removing wipe or use an icy washcloth.

Here is another trick you can do with the actual banana. Mash the fruit gently in a small bowl and add a quarter-sized amount of Vaseline. Place the mixture in the freezer for five minutes and then apply it under your eyes. Allow it to sit on your face for five minutes and then gently tissue off. Wrinkles, lines, and swelling will be visibly reduced, and your foundation and concealer will glide right on! Again, make certain you use a wipe for removal prior to putting on your makeup (a cold one works best)!

Doing either of these treatments can help reduce swelling, dark circles, and crepey skin, and can help reduce the appearance of wrinkles around the eyes because the peel and fruit of the banana contain natural firming fibers and anti-inflammatory extracts.

Cucumber Smooth Silhouette

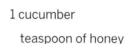

1 cucumber

teaspoon of honey

You've heard about chilling cucumber slices and placing them on puffy eyes, but that is not the main advantage you can obtain when harnessing this magical veggie for its beauty benefits. Here's another trick: First peel off the outer skin of the cucumber. Then identify your deepest wrinkles. Dab some honey on the area and then use the cucumber skin just like a Band-Aid and place it on top of the honey. Leave the cucumber on for about ten minutes and you'll see an almost instant plumping and rejuvenating effect.

Or you can try this: In the morning, puree the remaining cucumber and add it to a glass of fiber water (flavored or unflavored, which can easily be found in your grocery store) to give you those super-anti-inflammatory benefits. Continue to drink the water throughout the day. If you're putting on a skin-hugging outfit that night, stop hydrating one hour prior to getting dressed. At that time, any bloating in your stomach will be greatly reduced. In addition, drinking the water can also help remove some of the redness in your eyes, thereby making them appear whiter, so your beautiful natural color will pop and you will look healthy!

Singing in the Rain Shower

1 cheesecloth strip (large enough to completely cover your shower
    head and be held in place by a rubber band)
1 guava, cut and sliced
1 rosemary sprig
1/2 cucumber, cut and sliced
1 large rubber band

To maximize your skin care in the shower, take one cheesecloth strip and place the guava, rosemary, and cucumber inside. Wrap the bundle around a shower-head with a rubber band and let the treated water soak into your skin. Your shower pressure should be set on low to allow the maximum benefits to cascade over your whole body.

Another alternative is to wrap a few slices of cucumber, lemon, and lime in a piece of muslin or a clean dish towel. Drizzle in some honey or the liquid from a vitamin E capsule and secure the sack over the showerhead with a strong rubber band. Again, make sure your shower pressure is low, and you'll find that the citrus bundle will help soften your skin.

Soak It In

2 Alka-Seltzer tablets

1/2 gallon of milk

1 cup dry oatmeal

1/2 cup honey

If your skin takes a beating in the winter weather, or if you just want to help with cellulite, try using this recipe the next time you run a bath. Place the Alka-Seltzer tablets and milk into a tub of warm water. Before you get in, mix the oatmeal (it's a natural exfoliant and skin soother) and honey (which is a binder for the oatmeal and natural skin conditioner), then slather it on and rub it in from head to toe. Then get into the tub for a relaxing and skin-benefiting soak. By dropping the two tablets of Alka-Seltzer into the warm lactic acid bath, the combination will deeply hydrate, smooth, tone, brighten, and enlighten your skin. Add on a shea or coco butter moisturizer after you towel off, and your skin will feel comfortable and silky soft.

Spa Time During Gym Time

Did you know you can actually turn your gym into a spa by using beauty treatments to give your skin that healthy glow whether you're lifting weights or spinning on a bike? Here's how it works: Typically you're in the gym from forty-five minutes to an hour, and if you're clever, you can simultaneously use that as a time to treat your hair and skin as well. What I suggest to a lot of my clients is to apply a hair mask (such as a deep conditioner or anything found at your local drugstore) before you enter the gym, and then put your hair up in a ponytail during your workout. No one around you will know the difference, and when you're done at the gym, you'll have treated your hair. Then, for your face, while you work out, you can put on a clear antiaging or antiacne mask (or one for whatever skin type you have, such as a mask made with papaya and/or guava), and it will create a thin film that will keep the nutrients on your face. And because you sweat while you exercise, your pores will be open, so you'll get even more benefits from the mask. It's awesome! When you're done with your workout, you've treated your hair to look younger, healthier, and shinier, and your skin has actually had an hour's worth of a treatment that you may not typically have time to do at home. I also recommend you hydrate with nutrient-infused water, which will benefit your entire body from your head to your toes.

Another thing to do is to bring treated towels with you into the gym to use during your workout. I tell all my clients to take two workout towels with them: an untreated one for wiping off the backs of each of the different machines and yoga mats you use and a treated one that is saturated with a solution that's going to help your skin every time you touch it to your face.

To treat your towels, make sure they have been completely dried in a dryer at home. Then use an antibacterial solution with tea tree oil in it and spray the towel both on the front and the back. Remember to only use one of the towels to dab your face and use the second one to wipe off the gym equipment. You can also carry a small spray bottle to the gym (for example, the travel-sized bottles you can get at the drugstore) filled with that same solution and spray it on your face or your body periodically throughout your workout. When you exercise, your pores open up, your body is pumping out toxins, and your bloodstream is going much faster from any cardio you're doing, so your skin is going to take in all those wonderful ingredients and reap the benefits faster. So how often should you do this during your workout? I suggest that every time you take a sip of your water, you also lightly spray your face or use the towel that has been treated. By doing this, you are sneaking in an extra treatment at the gym.

Your gym bag can also be used to store your beauty arsenal. I suggest keeping antibacterial wipes in your bag because you'll want to get the bacteria off your hands after touching all the machines. I recommend that you have two headbands: one as a workout headband to absorb all the sweat and the other for after your workout. Spray this second headband with tea tree oil and place it around your hairline area where a lot of women tend to break out. Again, this is almost like a postworkout minitreatment!

Clever Celebrity Skin-Care Secrets

Despite what you may believe, most celebrities aren't naturally picture-perfect beautiful. Even they have tricks and rituals they use to keep their skin looking so sensationally screenworthy. Here are a few they've shared with me over the years:

"I wash my face at night before I go to bed, I change my pillowcase all the time neurotically, and I always wipe off my phone after I use it."

—*Mila Kunis*

"My girlfriend introduced me to her 'face diet' theory: 'If I can't eat it, I won't put it on my face.' I've always liked that."

—*Brittany Ishibashi*

"My tip is pretty basic. Just wash your face every morning and every night. Always moisturize."

—*Lucy Hale*

"When I actually focus and I take my proper vitamins and antioxidants and drink tons of water, my skin gets better 100 percent of the time. It always improves more so than doing anything else to my skin. I do experiments with my own skin, sometimes where I'll drink certain things or not drink certain things, take certain vitamins or not take certain vitamins, and it makes such a huge difference!"

—*Jayde Nicole*

"Using toner tightens pores. Tighter pores provide a fresher and younger look!"

—*Lynn Collins*

"Remove the stress in your life where you can, and if you can find a microdermabrasion peel, do it!"

—*Nancy O'Dell*

"I always use sunblock to protect my skin and prevent signs of aging, like wrinkles, skin discoloration, and all the other harmful effects of sun exposure. I also try to get a good amount of sleep."

—*Brooke Nevin*

6

Troubleshooting 101: Cravings, Cocktails, Confounding Convictions, and More

LIFE IS ALL ABOUT HAVING A GOOD TIME (and yes, being a bit serious at times too). But on occasion, we all slip up and may indulge a little too much or have insatiable cravings for things we know aren't at the top of the world's healthiest food-and-drinks list. As a result, when we give in and let loose, our skin may not be receiving the best care we can give it. But the good news is there are some fixes to help when we find ourselves behaving less than perfect.

And just remember, not every crazy skin-care rumor you've heard about is true, so your body may not be as doomed as you think. There's absolutely a road back to having healthy skin, and I'm ready to show you a new path to get there. Read on to find out what's true and what's false when it comes to taking care of that beautiful skin of yours.

Good News for Chocoholics

It's no surprise that chocolate is among the number one candies purchased in the United States (gummy bears and licorice also top the list). It's delicious, affordable, and hard to resist, but did you know it also has several health benefits? The darker the chocolate, the better it is. This is because cocoa (the main ingredient in chocolate) contains isoflavonoids, polyphenols, and cocoa bioferments, all of which raise the antioxidant levels in your body —not to mention your libido, according to some studies! Dark chocolate also contains vitamins D and E, as well as antioxidants, all of which are great for your skin and body.

However, the darker the chocolate, the more bitter it is. So if you don't necessarily like the taste of dark chocolate, try a bar that has a lower level of cocoa (you'll see the percentage of cocoa on the packaging), which will make it taste less bitter. Bars that have 60–90 percent cocoa are good options. If you want an even less bitter-tasting chocolate, go for the ones containing 50–60 percent cocoa. You are still getting a higher amount of cocoa bioferments and antioxidants than a processed milk chocolate bar. Just weigh the bitterness versus the sweetness level for yourself and decide

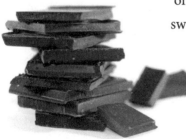

on the best percentage for you. I like sweeter-tasting chocolate, so I go with the lower cocoa content. Someone who likes a more bitter taste should go with a higher percentage of cocoa.

Drink It In

You need to drink adequate amounts of
water every day to keep your skin—as well
your entire system—healthy. Unfortunately, plain water may not be enough to
hold the right amount of moisture in your
body and lock it into your cells. Therefore,
I recommend supplementing your water
with nutrients that will help lock in the
moisture your body needs to function at its
most effective level. My BORBA-enhanced

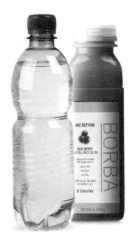

bottled water and crystallines are a good option for helping your
body hold on to moisture longer, but if it's not available to you, I
advise you to drink good-quality water that has been enhanced
with vitamins and minerals. To make sure you're getting the most
healthful enhanced water beverage, read the daily value content
listed on the label. If the label lists 10 percent in one serving, that's
not enough to give you any real benefit. In general, look for
waters that offer vitamins and minerals between 100% and 500%
of the daily value (or look for add-in powder packets with the
same potency). If you drink soda, it's best to do so in moderation.
For every twelve-ounce can of soda you drink, you should drink
a sixteen-ounce glass of water to offset the sugar content of the
soda and flush it out of your system faster. High levels of sugar in
your bloodstream slow down collagen production, which is not a
good thing for your skin.

If you are a soda drinker and are accustomed to having those jumbo twenty-ounce cups, my suggestion for you is to fill up the jumbo cup with ice and then put the soda in so the ice melts; as you drink, the ice will give you a little bit more liquid while it saturates into the soda. Also, sodas contain lots of acids, and over time they will challenge your beautiful white smile with corrosion. So no matter what beverage you decide to consume, it's always good to maintain a balanced soda-to-water ratio or caffeine-to-water ratio. For example, if you have a cup of coffee, make sure you have an 8-ounce glass of water as well. And, of course, always make certain that you have at least six 8-ounce glasses of water a day to keep your skin and body operating at top capacity. If you can't have six glasses and you still want to have your soda content each day, make certain that you also incorporate green leafy vegetables in your diet, because as we've already discussed, green leafy vegetables will actually help your body hold on to moisture internally a lot longer than just water alone.

Happy Hour

A glass of red or white wine is good for you in so many different ways (love those tannins, the polyphenols found in plants, oak barrels, and the seeds and stems of grapes, which can have a positive effect on your vascular health), and it's only about 100 calories in a single serving (about 4 ounces). But the dehydrating effects of wine are the same as that of vodka, which is even purer than a tannin-rich wine (and yes, a little bit of vodka can be a good thing!). So if you love your daily libation, make sure that before you drink, you hydrate your body, preferably with enhanced water, and after you drink, be sure to hydrate as well. Doing both together will replenish lost fluids and help you avoid having skin that looks tired and dried out. And, of course, you can always sip on one of my Borbatinis as a healthier alternative.

But let's say you do have one too many drinks. Fortunately, there are a few things you can to do reduce the physical after-effects (that puffiness and those dark or red eyes) from a night on the town. And it all starts before your head hits the pillow. Try these three simple steps as soon as you get home.

Step 1: Drinking enhanced water will help rehydrate and replenish your body. So the minute you take your keys out of the door, open a bottle and drink up! You need the skin-nourishing ingredients from things like lychee extract, green tea extract, vitamins K, E, and A, and papaya and guava extracts before that alarm goes off in the morning. Mixing one or two packets of BORBA Replenishing Lychee Fruit Antioxidant Crystalline Drink Mix with 16 ounces of water will definitely do the trick as well.

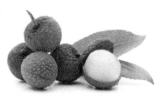

Step 2: Make sure you hydrate the exterior of your skin with a great moisturizer, even if you're too tired to remove your makeup and that's the only thing you have the energy to do. You'll be thanking me in the morning! Any cream or lotion will do, but an antiaging cream may be the best product to help you achieve that brighter and not-so-hungover look you're going for.

Step 3: Before you go to bed, make sure you eat something sweet to get your sugar levels up. Otherwise, it might just be a trip to cotton-mouth city for you! This is a time where putting a little sugar in your body isn't such a bad thing because it helps replace the sugar levels lost during your night out. This can help make sure your blood sugar levels don't drop too low in the middle of the night. You can always try snacking on my BORBA Omega-3 Citrus Bursts, calcium or fiber-rich chews, or fibrous fruits like nectarines, apples, or pears.

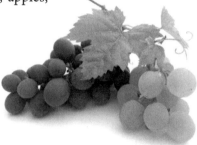

The next morning, be sure to continue drinking your enhanced water (definitely before downing your coffee!) and use a good eye cream to help reduce those dark circles under your peepers. It's also important to use a moisturizer on your entire body with ingredients such as sage leaf extract, lychee, or grape seed extract, which help promote long-term hydration for your skin. Other ingredients, such as bioferments in cocoa and aloe, can help maintain your skin's firmness.

And if you still feel like you need an extra dose of refreshment, try doing an at-home banana facial (see Chapter 5). It can perk up your tired eyes, firm up some of that loose skin, and give you a wide-awake look to mask your previous night's indulging!

Going on a Binge

You may not call it binge eating, but many of us do this without even realizing it. You don't eat for many hours and then when you finally do, you eat far too much and fill yourself up with foods that are less than healthy. A lot of people tend to binge when they're really happy, or sad, or tired from a long day at work. But binging is just not a good practice on so many levels and will be reflected in the way your body looks and feels. At the end of the day, it's all about controlling your consumption. If there's a big meal waiting for you and you feel like you're going to binge eat, have a small snack first. It really will make a difference in what you wind up putting into your body.

I used to overeat when I went for long periods without eating, so to keep myself from doing this, I keep a stash of soy bars, toasted soy nuts, blanched salt-free nuts, and dark chocolate pieces in my office. I also have the BORBA Slimming Chocolate Chews or BORBA Skin Balance Gummi Bears on hand, (which contain a lot of pectin). When pectin expands in your stomach, it makes you feel fuller faster. Because I consume these alternatives to junk food, my body now craves something healthier rather than something that is bad for me, like the cheese-flavored chips that I used to love so much! Try to keep nutritious snacks handy and you will gradually get your body accustomed to loving them.

Ravenous Rewards

Does this sound familiar? You work all day long and don't eat just because you're working so hard. I know I do that all the time, and while I'm going and going, I'll just drink coffee and my BORBA water. Then when I get everything done, that's when I reward myself with eating. And unfortunately, that's not a healthy thing to do, and there are plenty of men and women out there who do that far too often. They don't eat when they're hungry when they are supposed to. They don't eat those three meals or the five small meals a day that they're supposed to. Instead, they'll reward themselves by eating when things are done—like telling themselves they won't eat until they do what they need to do with their kids during their day and get everyone to bed. Or they won't eat until a big project at work is finished. But unfortunately, that pattern whacks out your whole metabolism. It whacks out your hydration levels, your skin, your muscle growth, and the tonality of your body. It whacks out everything.

So many of my clients in the entertainment world do this too. They tell themselves they won't eat until they memorize a portion of their scripts, or they won't go to the coffee shop until all of their errands are done and things like that. This is definitely *not* a healthy habit to keep! You must feed your body throughout the day for it to function properly, which will, of course, be reflected on the outside.

Bottom line—reward eating is not good. You have to reward yourself throughout the day to reward your skin—earn that beauty from the inside and out. I am guilty of doing this, so I had to recondition my mind throughout the day to reward my skin and reward my body to look and feel its best.

Eat and Drink Up ... on Schedule!

When your body is continually hydrated and fueled with nutritious foods and beverages, it will operate at maximum efficiency. This will help repair your skin faster regardless of your skin type or issue. Therefore, you should be grazing on small healthy snacks and meals and hydrating all day long on a fairly consistent schedule. Regulation is the key to everything. If you follow a schedule, you'll feel better overall. For example, have breakfast, lunch, and dinner and your snacks at approximately the same time every day. Also, have a set time to take your supplements (carry them with you if you're on the go). It's always a good idea to drink water when you wake up, before your first cup of coffee. If you don't consider yourself a big water drinker and turn to carbonated beverages instead, you will need to fortify your drinks throughout the day by drinking water infused with key nutrients.

Summer Skin

As everyone knows, to prevent a sunburn, you must wear sunblock—EVERY day! And since we're on the run all the time, try to use a physical block with elements of titanium dioxide and zinc oxide. The ingredients work immediately on contact with your skin so you don't have to wait for them to soak in before you head to the car or to the beach.

Look for a product that incorporates a full spectrum of UVA and UVB, which will give you carbon protection from the ozone and the environment, which helps avoid sunburns and the sun's harmful rays. Be certain to use a product that has a mattifying component (dimethicone and/or titanium dioxide, which are both natural skin mattifiers, and will be listed in the formula on the label) to keep skin looking healthy and not greasy.

However, if you've gotten sunburned, what should you do? Here are a few tips to help soothe your burn and decrease the damage to your skin:

☼ **Take a milk bath.** Fill your tub with cool water. Then add 1 gallon of milk (for that helpful vitamin D) and two Alka-Seltzer tablets to help immediately soothe irritation. Slowly add 12 to 24 ice cubes to the water as your body acclimates to the cool temperature. Slip into the bath and let the healing begin! Stay in for a minimum of 30 minutes to allow the lactic acid to penetrate your skin and then rinse off with cold or tepid water.

☼ **Sour cream is another at-home soother.** Slather a dollop of sour cream on the affected areas of your skin. Cover with an ice-cold washcloth for a few minutes and repeat until the stinging and burning dissipate. Rinse with cold or tepid water.

☼ **Yogurt can help too—the thicker the better!** Yogurt has the same soothing power as sour cream, but it is better for more sensitive skin types. So here's what you do. Take a freezer bag and fill it up with plain yogurt. Let it stand in the freezer for thirty minutes. Then take it out and puncture the front and back with a fork. Let that sit on the sunburned area and compress it with a cool towel (that also absorbs the excess dripping). That should do the trick! Rinse with cold or tepid water.

☼ **Take two large potatoes, chop them up, and toss them into a blender.** Add a tablespoon of honey for skin adhesion and press "puree." Coat your sunburned area with this paste and you'll start to feel relief within minutes. Rinse off in the shower with cold or tepid water.

☼ **How about them apples?** Green Granny Smith apples have higher anti-inflammatory agents than red apples, so take one green apple, chop it up, add a tablespoon of honey for skin adhesion, and toss everything into a blender. Press "puree" and then coat the sunburned area with the fruity concoction for a fast and calming sensation. Rinse off in the shower with cold or tepid water.

☼ **You can also try chilling your aloe vera or anti-inflammatory moisturizer or cream in the refrigerator for an hour before you apply it on your skin.** The sheer coolness will help relieve the sensation of burning and will help to calm redness and inflammation.

☼ **If you have a sunburn, keep your skin hydrated throughout the day.** Any skin atomizer will be a welcome skin quencher, and continuously spritzing it onto your skin will help lock in moisture.

☼ **Stay out of extreme temperatures.** Going into a very cold environment after you get sunburned could feel very uncomfortable, so ease your damaged skin into a comfortable temperature with gradual steps.

Crackly Skin Be Gone: Wondrous Winter Care

As winter approaches, the weather gets colder, and unfortunately, your skin gets dryer. Therefore, you need to alter your skin care to find the right combination to keep your body moisturized and healthy. Gentle cleaning helps remove the daily impurities and dead skin that can build up and cause blemishes and blackheads, but here are a few other things you can do to manage this seasonal situation.

❄ **Facial creams rich in antioxidants help repair the damage caused by winter weather.** Tip: Apply your eye cream to the skin around your mouth. This helps diminish the appearance of fine lines and the peeling of dry skin.

❄ **Even during the winter, putting SPF on your skin is a great idea.** Although the sun may be hiding, the rays that reflect off the snow and peek through the clouds are just as damaging as the summer sun.

❄ **Exfoliate one to two times a day to dissolve the buildup on your face and exfoliate your body twice a week.** This gives you a deeper cleanse, which allows your skincare products to work more effectively.

Skin Rx when Traveling

Just because you're not at home doesn't mean you have to abandon your beauty routine. You can still look and feel your best no matter if you're on the road, in the air, or chilling at a hotel in a new city. Don't be tempted to stray from your traditional products because of a travel-sized impulse purchase. Even temporarily switching to a different brand or product can mess with your skin. I always say to forgo potential irritation and adverse reactions by investing in TSA-size tubes for your tried-and-true products. Your skin will thank you.

I have a secret tip for soothing the dry skin we all get when flying: Mix your hand cream with a little hand sanitizer. It not only departs dryness, but the protective barrier allows you to feel like you can touch things around you a few times without massive consequences. And of course, that high altitude never fails to cause dehydration. To avoid a parched, dull complexion, prep yourself internally and externally before you board the plane by loading up on vitamins E and A (for skin moisture), vitamin C, zinc (for skin resilience), and at least a liter of water. The water will help the vitamins circulate in your system for a longer period and help them absorb easier. And speaking of water, absolutely power hydrate on any flight that is more than forty-five minutes. If you can, try to bring a bottle of water with you on the plane (purchased inside the airport, of course) to sip from throughout your flight, just in case the drink cart isn't readily available.

Another alternative if you don't want to bring the water bottle with you is filling up on pectin-rich foods like peaches, apples, or oranges.

So how can you tell if your skin is dehydrated during your long flight? Since the skin underneath your eyes is very thin, if it starts to appear a bit sunken in or dry, that's one of the telling signs of dehydration. Keep an ultramoisturizing eye cream on board and apply a thin layer every two hours to ensure the plane ride and landing end smoothly for your eyes.

Here are a few more airborne skin-saving suggestions:

- **Try to get your beauty sleep.** It's a fact that we sleep better when it's dark, so on your next flight, pack a freshly washed sleeping mask to cover your eyes. Also, germs can hide everywhere on a plane, so be sure to pack a clean pillowcase if you plan on using an airline-supplied pillow.

- **Freshen up the right way!** The water in a plane's lavatory is great for washing your hands, but if you wash your face with it, your face could become dried out from the minerals in the water. I always recommend taking a bottle of purified water with you (purchased after you go through security) to wash your face on a plane.

- **I have a lot of celebrity clients who are worried what their makeup will look like when they get off a flight (you never know where those paparazzi are hiding!).** I always have them wear the basics (eyeliner, mascara, blush, and a light dusting of foundation) and lock those in with an antiaging serum. Not only does their makeup look natural, but pressing in the serum over the makeup helps the makeup last longer too (up to eight hours without reapplying).

In order to keep your skin safe from any free radicals or bacteria hiding in a hotel room, I suggest bringing an antibacterial spray with you that includes skin-protecting ingredients. The first thing you should always do when you enter your room is pull down the comforter and mist the antibacterial spray over the sheets and pillowcases, lounging chairs, and even the robes hanging in the closet. Not only are you helping to fortify the defense against bacteria, but everything that touches your skin will be infused with skin-care ingredients to make you look and feel younger! But if you're carrying your suitcase onto the plane and can't bring the spray with you, try packing a TSA-approved travel spray bottle (less than 3 ounces) filled with a tea tree and water mixture. It will work just as well on your hotel linens.

The Truth Behind Skin-Care Myths and Misconceptions

Misconceptions are everywhere and exist for every skin type. There are misconceptions about how often you need to change your pillowcases and your sheets (see Chapter 3). There are misconceptions about using bar soap instead of a gel cleanser. There have been misconceptions about certain foods actually causing signs of aging, or acne, or cellulite, or weight challenges (see Chapter 4). These misguided concepts are everywhere, but knowing the facts will help you muddle through and come out on the other side armed with the skin-saving truth.

Myth: **Greasy foods and chocolate are the cause of acne.**

Fact: Can you imagine life without an occasional side of fries or a candy bar? Not me! There is no scientific evidence firmly linking acne to poor food choices in the fast-food lane. One of the main causes of acne (outside of your environment and the weather) is hormones, which cause oil buildup in the skin. You may want to cut back on pizza and candy bars for other important health reasons, but eating dark chocolate can actually be good for you (see Chapter 6)! Of course, healthy foods, and all the best nutrients nature has to offer, can help every cell in your body to be radiant—especially your face—so have the healthy stuff as often as you can. But indulging in those tempting bad-for-you treats once in a while is totally okay by me. Just be smart about it.

Myth: **Not drinking enough water will cause you to lose the elasticity in your skin.**

Fact: Yes, water is extremely important in maintaining healthy skin. But it's not just about the H_2O. It's also about eating the right foods, like leafy green vegetables, which will help you hold on to moisture longer than just drinking water (see Chapter 4). Adding moisture-rich foods to your diet will actually keep your cells hydrated longer so you'll look more youthful, with skin that's tauter and less dry and cracked.

Myth: **Taking long, hot showers will help keep your skin moisturized.**

Fact: Not true—in fact, it may have the opposite effect. If you use water that is too hot on your skin for longer than three minutes, you can actually dry it out and cause challenges such as eczema, psoriasis, redness, and breakouts! So shortening those showers or lowering the heat level may help solve some of your dry skin dilemmas.

Myth: **Lipstick doesn't have any negative side effects.**

Fact: Actually, it might! You work so hard to get the proper amount of antioxidants into your body all day long, but if you are wearing unnatural petroleum-based lipsticks, you are ingesting the unnatural chemicals and preservatives all day long, which may actually hinder the effects of those antioxidants going through your bloodstream! By switching to lipstick with more natural ingredients, you will get the full benefits of the anti-oxidants you're eating.

Myth: **If you have sensitive skin, you can't drink red wine because it's going to make you blush.**

Fact: That is simply not true. If you're a drinker with sensitive skin and you want to have a glass of wine or a beer without that rosy glow, you can take an anti-inflammatory agent before you drink. You can do this by eating a serving of goji berries, apples, spinach, almonds, or other anti-inflammatory foods before you head out for the night. Even taking an over-the-counter anti-inflammatory medication, like ibuprofen, in advance can help and will help keep you looking refreshed and rested. So don't fear—just because you have problem skin doesn't mean you can't have that relaxing glass of red wine once in a while. And besides, those tannins are quite good for you!

Myth: **Ethnicity always determines your skin type.**

Fact: No, it doesn't! Ethnicity determines your genetic makeup, but other factors will play a much bigger role in what happens with your skin over your lifetime. Any ethnicity can trick you into thinking that you might have problems. You may think that just because you have a certain skin color, you will automatically ash up or that you are definitely going to have major follicular problems like ingrown hairs. But that may never happen to you. Every human body is different, and you need to look at both your body and your environment, not just your ethnicity, to solve your skin problems. It's a combination of everything. Weather could be a major factor. If your skin is oily, it might be because you live in a humid climate and not because of your race. If you are always parched, it might be from living in a dry climate. It could be about your diet. It could be about the products you're using. It could be how hot or cold the water is on your skin. The bottom line is that you need to pay less attention to your ethnicity and spend more time figuring out how to work with your environment instead of the environment working against you.

Myth: **If your skin is oily or breaks out easily, you can't use a moisturizer.**

Fact: Of course you can . . . and you definitely *should*! All skin types need moisture, so omitting that step from your skin-care routine will only cause more problems. In fact, a water-based moisturizer is an important part of keeping the skin cells healthy and preventing dead skin cell buildup. Most moisturizers are made with ingredients that won't clog pores or cause more acne, but just to be safe, try one that's oil free. And for those of you who have oily skin, try products that contain antiaging ingredients or SPF (see more about this in Chapter 2).

Myth: Expensive products are better for your skin than cheaper ones.

Fact: Absolutely not! The cost of a product does not correlate to how effective it is. In fact, that inflated price most likely reflects the item's marketing and elaborate packaging rather than the skin-care product itself. You actually can find the same active ingredients that do the "magical" trick in pricey products in much less expensive drugstore brands. You just need to inspect the labels and become an expert at what to look for (see Chapter 2). As long as the right ingredients are in the product you're using, the price tag won't make a difference.

Myth: Popping pimples will help them go away faster.

Fact: If you pop a pimple, it may look less noticeable for a short time, but you're doing more damage than good. When you squeeze the blemish, you can actually push bacteria, oil, and dead skin cells further into the skin, which in turn can cause additional swelling and redness. And often, it will end up leaving a red mark or scar where the pimple was that can last for weeks or even months! So your best bet is to let pimples be or use topical products to decrease their appearance while you use internal methods to reduce your acne.

However, if you are going to extract a pimple, there are a few delicate steps you need to take to avoid damaging your skin. If a pimple is very tender, red, or painful, *leave it alone*. The more blood that is near the surface of the skin means the greater chance an extraction will turn into a bruise or a scar. If the pimple is white, small, and is not sore, it is a pustule that can be extracted fairly easily. Some people prefer to do extractions by hand, and a disinfected extraction tool can also be used, but if it is used with too much pressure, it could definitely cause a bruise or a scar. Clean, sanitized fingertips with clean fingernails are the safest, most effective way for beginners, or you can use the edges of two cotton swabs.

- First, a pimple should be examined before any pressure is applied to determine if the pustule is mature enough to extract. The white area of a pimple is pus, which is a part of the body's immune defense. Extraction will release the pus and any excess blood that is built up in the pimple.
- Next, once the pimple is confirmed to be a pustule (has a white head) that is close to the surface of the skin and is not tender, extraction may begin by applying pressure around the white area with the index fingers of your hands, pushing both sides of the pustule together until the skin breaks and the pus is released.
- Last, the area should be immediately cleaned with mild soap and water to avoid infection.

However, if the bump is of a different consistency than a whitehead, it may be a cyst. A cyst usually has a hard center and stays in your skin. To heal, you would need to get a cortisone injection or have it cut out by a professional, which can leave a scar. So the fast and simple rule is this: if you can feel a hard center, go to a professional.

Myth: Tanning is harmless.

Fact: Any type of tanning—in the sun or in a tanning bed—will expose your skin to ultraviolet light (UVA or UVB), which is one of the major causes of premature skin aging and can cause major skin damage. Your risk of cancer and other skin disorders increases, and you can wind up with more wrinkles, age spots, and even skin discoloration. If you really desire that sun-kissed glow, try one of the numerous bronzers, self-tanning lotions, or creams that are in your local drugstore. You'll look just as tan without any of the harmful side effects!

Myth: Touching your face too much causes wrinkles.

Fact: Not true. Wrinkles are caused by things like too much sun exposure, smoking, squinting, and even smiling or frowning repeatedly over time. It's not from touching your face or from having dry skin. Rubbing your mug can cause irritation, but it won't cause you to have wrinkles. The reason for this is simple: you're not always rubbing or touching your face in the same place or continuously for long periods of time, which is what would need to happen in order to leave a permanent mark. Unfortunately, you can't completely prevent wrinkles from forming (it's a combination of genetic and environmental factors), but you can do things to reduce their appearance and slow down the aging process, like fortifying your body with antioxidants, reducing free-radical damage, and staying out of the sun. When it comes to skin-care products to use, the key ingredients for helping with this issue are retinol peptides, which are small proteins that stimulate collagen production and increase skin cell turnover. They can be purchased over the counter or through your doctor if you need a higher-strength prescription.

When Celebrities Say "Aagh!" Rather than "Aha!"

Even some of the most recognized and most glamorous celebrities in the world have skin issues. But they have the added pressure of being photographed by the paparazzi every time they leave their house and of being filmed every day when they go to work. Looking pretty on-screen and offscreen isn't always as easy as it seems. That's why they call it "Movie Magic"! Here are a few of the biggest skin complaints from some of my celebrity clients:

"I am fully aware of when I have a breakout on my face. So when that happens at work and I'm going to be on camera, I have to give the heads-up to my director of photography, and then they have to use extra lighting and use more lighting boards to help conceal those flaws. It's the worst."

—*Mila Kunis*

"Theater makeup really did me in! Caking it on seven days a week and working under hot lights translated into breakout city and dryness. Blech!"

—*Brittany Ishibashi*

"I've had frequent breakouts because of my age and the line of work I'm in. Because looking good is almost a requirement, I needed to take some extra steps, like facials, to help."

—*Lucy Hale*

"When I was in my late teen years, my acne was awful. I had to go on Accutane. The acne I had was terribly embarrassing! You never think about your skin when it looks good, but when it's bad, it's hard to think about anything else."

—*Lynn Collins*

"I have a job that keeps me on the go, so I deal with stress on a daily basis. And also because of my work, I have heavy makeup caked on my face every day for hours and hours, which makes it more difficult to keep my skin glowing and clear."

—*Nancy O'Dell*

Listening to Your Inner Voice

Whether you're at home, traveling, or even just trying to keep up with a hectic on-the-go schedule, it's extremely important to listen to your body and your inner voice, because only *you* truly know when something isn't quite right with your system. Watch out for those red flags. If you are feeling a little bit off, like maybe you feel a little dehydrated, or your eyes feel a little dry, you notice more redness in your eyes, or notice that your eyes are less white, do something about it. Maybe you notice that your nail beds are less pink or your nails aren't as strong as they once were. Maybe you're noticing more dry patches on your skin or your hair is a little bit duller. If anything you notice is a little more off than normal, these things are indicators that your body is transitioning into something and you might want to change your routine to get yourself back in sync.

It's really important for you to be in tune with your body so you will notice when anything, even something small, begins to change. If you're getting dandruff, that is a sign of dehydration as well as a sign that your sebaceous glands are drying up. It could also be a sign that you are moving from perimenopause to menopause, signaling that it's time to speak with your doctor about what's going on and how to treat your body accordingly.

If you've never gotten eczema or psoriasis patches, but now you're getting them, one of the triggers might be stress. That stress is showing up initially by your eczema and psoriasis (which manifests as itchy, raised bumps on your skin), but soon after that, it could show up as major acne, cystic acne, pronounced crow's feet on your face, crepey skin, or dark circles under your eyes. There's time to fix the problem from the inside out, so listen to what your body is telling and showing you!

If you're going to be moving from one place to another, you may be headed for climate changes, elevation changes, or seasonal changes, so you need to prep your skin ahead of time. Just like you prep yourself for a test, you need to do that with your skin, and you need to acclimate your body to the climate, elevation level, or stress level you are about to encounter.

Bottom line is that by really listening and tuning in to your body, you'll be able to prevent and fix problems with your skin before or right when they happen, which in turn will help you keep yourself as healthy as possible. You know yourself the best, and if your inner voice is telling you something is off or is changing, it probably is!

7

Who Knew?
Insider Tips and Tricks

T HIS CHAPTER IS FULL OF INSIDER beauty tips and the most frequently asked questions I hear about everything from your eyes to your thighs. I'll answer some of the questions many of you are wondering about but have always been afraid to ask, and hopefully the answers will be the ones you've been searching for.

Radiant Eyes

Don't miss out on the opportunity to let your eyes radiate your inner beauty. Here are a few tips for putting your best eyes forward whenever and wherever:

- Eye cream should be called "eye candy." Your eyes can become damaged from dryness due to a lack of oil glands around them. To reverse the dryness, fine lines, and wrinkles that can show up, use a good moisturizing eye cream every morning and evening.

- Your ring finger, which is your weakest finger, can exert just the right amount of strength to be used as an ideal application tool. Using your ring finger to put on your eye cream will produce a gentle pressure that can maximize the overall results of applying products around the eyes.

- Use your refrigerator to enhance your eye cream results. A simple rule of physics is that cold contracts molecules and heat expands them. This is why cold weather deflates tires and balloons. Why is this important? It's as true for your car tires and balloons as it is for you. Putting your eye cream in the fridge for a few minutes before applying it to your eyes will help reduce puffiness quicker than if you use it at room temperature.

- Apply a thin layer of petroleum jelly over your favorite eye cream before bed. This will trap in moisture to plump up delicate skin overnight, keeping your eyes constantly conditioned, and by morning, your puffy eyes will be gone!

- Sunglasses can do more than just make you look cool; they protect your eyes. Wearing proper eyewear every time you're outside or in your car can help reduce the squinting that can cause fine lines. It also gives you a healthy excuse to rock those expensive sunglasses you bought!

Here are a few eye questions I always get asked:

Q: Why do I get dark circles under my eyes?

A: The reason the skin surrounding eyes can get so dark is due to something that almost no one is immune from: ruptured capillaries in the delicate layer of skin above the bones surrounding the eye sockets. As we age, or when we get ill, the pressure that aging skin can have on the capillaries can cause them to rupture. This happens because the skin is resting right on top of the actual bone, and there is very little cushion left to soften the impact. There are a few things you can do to prevent, or at least severely reduce, the appearance of these dark distracters:

* You can nourish, moisturize, and rest.
* As for products, using an oxygenating facial mask will help protect your skin and alleviate some of the pressure resulting from environmental and physical causes.
* You might also want to try adding a moisturizing SPF to your daily skin-care routine to help slow down the aging process.

Q: Do you have any at-home tricks for getting rid of dark circles or puffiness under my eyes?

A: Absolutely! There are a few things you can do to revitalize dark or puffy eyes.

* First, try to get a bit more sleep at night. Also, try to set aside thirty minutes each day to relax or meditate and try to enjoy some "me" time.

* If that doesn't help, you can try placing cold cucumber slices over your eyes for fifteen minutes before you leave the house. Or, for more lasting effects, as I've mentioned before, place your eye cream in the refrigerator and then apply it chilled in the morning. The combination of cold and delivery of antioxidants to your problem areas should help to make an immediate, as well as a longer-term, solution for fixing your dilemma.

* Last, my favorite quick fix for dark circles or puffiness is to put an ice cube on the roof of your mouth and hold it there with your tongue. The cold will literally help draw down the puffiness underneath the eye area. In a few minutes, you'll look more refreshed and awake!

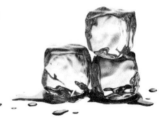

Abolishing Acne

Q: **What's the fastest and healthiest remedy for acne?**

A: There are a few healthy things you can do to help keep skin clear of blemishes.

* First, make sure you drink plenty of fluids during the day. By doing so, you will help to flush toxins from your body.

* Second, use a cleanser that has the ability to keep your skin balanced and helps prevent pores from clogging up.

Look for a cleanser that contains ingredients such as zinc and vitamins A, B, and E.

* If you're looking for a completely natural remedy, try placing either tea tree oil or superfoods like tomatoes, honey, or cucumber slices directly onto your acne. Tea tree oil has natural anti-bacterial properties that can help with the pain, redness, and swelling of the inflammation of your acne. The acid in tomatoes will slightly soften your skin, and its vitamin A will help your skin stay elastic, which in turn will prevent more clogs from forming. Honey is actually one of the best natural acne-fighting ingredients because it kills the bacteria that cause acne in the first place. And finally, the skin of cucumber slices has a ton of vitamins and other nutrients that will help to not only get rid of acne, but will also help your skin be more resilient to prevent future acne problems.

Q: I have lots of whiteheads all over my forehead. I've tried so many different products! How do I get my beautiful skin back?

A: Whiteheads are typically caused by oil and dirt that get stuck in pores that are unable to drain, causing bacteria to form. It's important that you wait until they're fully grown before removing them, as popping them can cause scarring or a larger infection. However, you can prevent further whiteheads from growing by making sure you cleanse often (two times a day). You can use a facial cleanser with benzoyl peroxide, which will help kill bacteria (but could be harsh on sensitive skin), sulfur, or salicylic acid, which can help to exfoliate your skin and open the pores and prevent blockage.

Q: **Can I use mineral and liquid makeup together, or will that make my skin break out?**

A: Many products out there are "noncomedogenic," meaning that they won't clog pores and cause acne or cystic acne. Aside from using only products that are noncomedogenic, special application steps should be followed to further help avoid potential problems when combining mineral and liquid makeup. These include:

* To make sure mineral makeup goes on evenly and looks more natural, put your liquid makeup on first.
* Always apply liquid makeup as a thin layer with a sponge. Avoid overly saturating a specific area as this can cause irritation and can cause pores to become blocked.
* When the product has dried, it's safe to run a dry sponge over your entire face to wipe off any excess.
* Once the liquid makeup is dry and applied to your liking, the dusting of mineral makeup can begin. Again, caking

READER/CUSTOMER CARE SURVEY

HEFG

We care about your opinions! Please take a moment to fill out our online Reader Survey at **http://survey.hcibooks.com.**

As a **"THANK YOU"** you will receive a **VALUABLE INSTANT COUPON** towards future book purchases

as well as a **SPECIAL GIFT** available only online! Or, you may mail this card back to us.

First Name   MI.   Last Name

Address   City

State   Zip   Email

1. Gender
☐ Female   ☐ Male

2. Age
☐ 8 or younger   ☐ 13-16
☐ 9-12   ☐ 17-20   ☐ 21-30
☐ 31+

3. Did you receive this book as a gift?
☐ Yes   ☐ No

4. Annual Household Income
☐ under $25,000
☐ $25,000 - $34,999
☐ $35,000 - $49,999
☐ $50,000 - $74,999
☐ over $75,000

5. What are the ages of the children living in your house?
☐ 0 - 14   ☐ 15+

6. Marital Status
☐ Single
☐ Married
☐ Divorced
☐ Widowed

7. How did you find out about the book?
(please choose one)
☐ Recommendation
☐ Store Display
☐ Online
☐ Catalog/Mailing
☐ Interview/Review

8. Where do you usually buy books?
(please choose one)
☐ Bookstore
☐ Online
☐ Book Club/Mail Order
☐ Price Club (Sam's Club, Costco's, etc.)
☐ Retail Store (Target, Wal-Mart, etc.)

9. What subject do you enjoy reading about the most?
(please choose one)
☐ Parenting/Family
☐ Relationships
☐ Recovery/Addictions
☐ Health/Nutrition
☐ Christianity
☐ Spirituality/Inspiration
☐ Business Self-help
☐ Women's Issues
☐ Sports

10. What attracts you most to a book?
(please choose one)
☐ Title
☐ Cover Design
☐ Author
☐ Content

FOLD HERE

Comments

on or overly saturating a specific area can cause irritation, so be sure to use light, even strokes while applying.

* And of course, make sure your brushes and sponges are clean. You should lightly clean your brushes every day and intensely clean them in a disinfectant about twice a week. Sponges should be used once and tossed. Also, beware of double-dipping: a palette similar to a painter's palette can be used to mix makeup and will help avoid cross-contamination.

Q: **I have very fair skin, which is somewhat dry and prone to breakouts. I need a high SPF, but a light moisturizer. What should I do?**

A: You can never have too much SPF. You can use either a chemical or topical variety, but if you have sensitive skin, use a topical sunscreen, such as titanium dioxide. Those products should not cause you to break out and will help to moisturize as well.

Q: **Would you recommend applying moisturizer to acne-prone skin at night versus the morning, since skin loses more moisture at night?**

A: All skin requires moisture, and acne-prone skin is no different. Moisturizers aren't the bad guys when it comes to acne. As mentioned earlier, acne is caused by a number of pore-clogging factors, including hormones, hygiene, and diet.

If you have acne, especially if you are on topical or ingestible meds for acne, you want to be sure you keep as moisturized as possible to avoid damaging the outer layers of the dermis. My suggestion would be to use a moisturizer that is non-comedogenic with a superhydrating ingredient like argan oil both day and night, along with any acne prescriptions you're using.

Agonizing over Aging Skin

Q: I'm twenty, and I was wondering if I should be using antiaging products yet?

A: The one thing you should know about antiaging regimens is that it is **never too early** to start! I'm serious. Aging begins for most of us somewhere in our teens, but most of us don't start to think about it until well into our late thirties or sometimes early forties. So when it finally matters, there is so much more damage that needs to be dealt with to recapture a youthful appearance. So start now and you'll be thanking yourself in the future.

Q: What is the number one most important product I should be using for antiaging and what are your thoughts on Retin-A?

A: In my opinion, the number one most important product you should use for antiaging is a moisturizer with SPF protection. It's amazing how much environmental damage we expose ourselves to each day, such as dry air, the sun's UVA/B rays, and pollution, when we don't use SPF. As for my thoughts on Retin-A, it can be an effective skin treatment if you do not have sensitive skin. But I will warn you, it does have a few side effects, such as burning, dry skin, itching, peeling, redness, and stinging, which makes it unpleasant for some who use it.

Q: **What can I do to get rid of dark spots and make my complexion more radiant and even-toned?**

A: Dark spots are often quite difficult to treat. The easiest thing to do for dark spots is to prevent the causes of dark spots before they begin. The best way to do this is by protecting the skin with some form of moisturizing sunblock. I should also note before addressing how to remove them that once you begin treating dark spots, it's very important to apply moisturizing sunblock protection forever after, or the darkness will return. So how do you treat dark spots? There are two things that should be done before protecting your skin. First, use a deep exfoliator, preferably one that's a chemical peel, and second, apply a skin brightener to hasten the lightening. To get the even tone, you'll need to exfoliate the entire area surrounding the dark spots so that the skin can repair itself as a whole and not just in scattered portions.

Obnoxiously Oily Skin

Q: I have really oily skin and have tried lots of products, but they don't seem to work. So I use rubbing alcohol, which seems to clean out my pores, leaving my skin oil free for a little while. Is this a good idea?

A: No! Putting alcohol on your skin to get rid of oil is like putting a fire out by throwing gasoline on it! While you may have had oily skin to begin with and the alcohol will remove all of the oil on your skin, it creates the never-ending oily-skin headache you're experiencing. Alcohol robs your body of the natural oil levels it needs to stay hydrated and tells your body you need to produce even more oil at an even faster and more copious rate to repair the imbalance you're creating. Oil is a very, very necessary ingredient for healthy skin. The trick is to get the oil level at just the right amount. From what your question infers, you've been using products that also dry your skin to levels that tell your body to create more oil. Products with benzoyl peroxide will certainly dry out your skin, and so will salicylic acid, which are both common ingredients in acne and oily skin care. Quite a catch-22, right?

This is the same problem I faced when I was growing up, and this is partly what led me to ultimately create my own line of skin-care products. You want to find products that keep your skin moisturized, won't strip the necessary oil levels needed, and will help to create a blemish-free complexion.

My recommendation for you is to try some of those products (or any product you find in your price range with similar ingredients) and add a fortified water to your diet. A clear complexion awaits!

Dealing with Dry Skin

Q: I just moved from an ocean city to one in the mountains, and now my skin is dry and I've been breaking out. What should I do?

A: The problems you're experiencing with your skin are likely due to the change in elevation. Higher altitudes can cause dry skin issues, along with a host of other issues (chapped lips, swollen feet, and so on). The most convenient thing you could do—and probably the best preventative measure—would be to drink fortified drinks that are specifically designed for dry skin issues (such as my Replenishing Lychee Fruit Skin Balance Water or Crystallines). If you're also experiencing chapped lips, you can try a balm or gloss that is rich in natural moisturizing oils like almond, coconut, sunflower, apricot, or peppermint, which will help protect your skin. Finally, if you already have dry skin damage, you can look for products that have a dimethicone level set at 5 percent and that are guaranteed to soften and moisturize dry skin.

Decreasing Discoloration

Q: How can I keep my skin from looking discolored?

A: To avoid skin that looks discolored, ditch your potentially streaky foundation and even out your skin tone with a tinted primer instead (a primer is a cosmetic designed for smoothing out the fine lines on your face to prepare it for applying makeup). It's the goof-proof route to a natural-looking, healthy glow. Plus, it will help your makeup stay put all day long!

Perfecting Problematic Pores

Q: I have massively huge pores and no matter what I try, I can't seem to find any facial care regimen that will help me with clearing them out and closing them up. What can I do?

A: I know how difficult it is to find products that work the way you need them to. So, I'm going to give you a few ingredients that will help you find a solution for large pores that are difficult to keep clear. Look for products that contain between 0.5–1 percent salicylic acid or 2.5–5 percent glycolic or lactic acid. These ingredients will help to exfoliate your skin, allowing for new skin with greater elasticity. This will help make your pores appear smaller.

Q: I recently developed a combination of clogged pores, breakouts, and very dry, flaky skin. What can I do to help both problems?

A: You should start with an exfoliation process. However, since your pores are also getting clogged with breakouts, I think the best thing you can do with your exfoliation treatment is to also reduce the size of your pores. Exfoliators with salicylic, glycolic, or lactic acid will help to reduce the size of your pores. In addition, vitamins A and C can also help to tighten the appearance of your skin. You can also try my 4-in-1 Cleansing Treatment—not only does it help to exfoliate dry skin and reduce the size of pores, but it also provides gentle moisturizing qualities.

Q: **Oil-control products dry out my skin, and the rich ones clog my pores. What should I do?**

A: This is a common problem many people face when using oily skin products and here's why. They're filled with acids, which by nature are dehydrating, and without proper moisturizing dry skin can occur. Benzoyl peroxide is another culprit for creating dry skin, and if possible, it should be paired with something to moisturize your skin after you apply it. So the easiest thing you can do is make sure your products will moisturize in conjunction with its oil-fighting properties. Sulfur-based oil-reducing skin-care products can certainly fit the bill. If your current product doesn't moisturize, you should think about adding another product designed solely for moisturizing, to be applied after you're finished with your oily skin treatment. When I tried to fix my blemish problems, I came up with a solution of using cotton fiber, which works to both reduce the appearance of blemishes and moisturize, leaving my skin feeling soft.

Concerns at Every Age

Skin problems and issues can change with age, so it's important to recognize the steps you should be taking year after year as you journey through life. The one thing you should do at every age is make sure your body is properly nourished to keep it as young-looking and healthy as possible for as long as possible. However, no matter how old or young you are, there are certain things that can make your skin go from fab to frightening in no time. In addition to the misuse of topical products or poor facial treatments (which can be detrimental to maintaining a healthy-looking and attractive completion), here is a list of hazards that can make your skin age more quickly:

- Dehydration
- Free radicals (from pollution, dirty filters, etc.)
- Hormone depletion
- Improper nutrition
- Lack of exercise
- Lack of sleep
- Medication/drugs
- Negative attitude, lifestyle
- Overindulgence of alcohol
- Overindulgence of caffeine
- Smoking

- Stress
- Vitamin deficiency

The good news is that fixing any or all of these problems before they get out of hand will help you and your skin look and feel healthier and keep people guessing when it comes to your real age! Read on for some important tips.

In Your Twenties

You still have that youthful glow and may feel like your body is invincible. But now is really the time you should start taking care of your skin so it doesn't experience damage in the future. It's all about sun protection. Using sunscreen is the single most important step to maintaining healthy skin over time. It's an investment in how you will look in your forties and fifties. Start to use a good moisturizer and light, thin, lotionlike eye cream (versus a thicker, heavy cream) too.

And at this stage of your life, there are a few skin issues that will most likely be popping up (no pun intended). The first issue you might come across is blackheads, which are clogged pores caused by a buildup of debris, oil, and dead skin cells. When they are open, the oxygen in the air turns them black. Fortunately, they can be exfoliated or extracted, so these unsightly blemishes won't be around for long (be sure to read "Exfoliate to Radiate" in Chapter 3 and the section about extracting pimples in Chapter 6). The second issue you might have is whiteheads, which occur when oil and dead skin are trapped beneath the surface of your skin and aren't exposed to air. The best way to remove them is by lancing them open and extracting what's inside. Of course, it's always best to have a professional do it to reduce the risk of scarring, so please consult your esthetician or dermatologist first.

Last, at this age, skin dehydration can be a definite dilemma. It happens when there is a lack of water in your body caused by overexertion and exercise or not eating healthy. It can also occur if you use the wrong topical agent or ingest dehydrating drinks such as caffeine or alcohol. The solution is easy—drink water, water, and more water. It's as simple as that!

In Your Thirties

Once you turn the big 3-0, you may feel that urge to start examining every inch of your skin, and that isn't such a bad idea. It's not too late for prevention, but now you may need to add on more treatments. Use eye cream to protect against excessive laugh lines and crow's feet. Use a mask to brighten your face and reduce the look of fine lines and wrinkles a minimum of twice a week and also use an exfoliant to remove dull skin every day (once or twice depending on your skin's sensitivity).

At this stage of the game, sun damage can begin to cause collagen and elastin breakdown, pigmentation, and possibly cancer on your body. So look closely at your skin and start your prevention with the use of a high SPF sunscreen. And here's a good tip: most people don't apply sunscreen as directed on the bottle, so always look for the higher numbered sunscreen, because the higher the better for protection if you are not using it correctly.

During these years, a skin issue that may become a concern is enlarged pores. This happens when oil and debris get trapped in the follicles and your skin expands, causing elasticity loss in that area. See the Q & A section of this chapter for suggestions of ways to help close them up, or you can try one of my at-home spa masks (see Chapter 5).

Two other issues that you should be on the lookout for at this age are erythema and seborrhea. Erythema is a redness caused by inflammation, overstimulation, not enough topical moisture protection, and genetic factoring. Seborrhea is oiliness of the skin caused by overstimulation of washing, toning, or wiping of the epidermis. Both conditions can be quelled by eating different foods specific to helping with these conditions (see Chapter 4) or by altering your skin-care methods to decrease the irritation to your body. Some suggestions in Chapter 5 may help as well.

In Your Forties

Some people say forty is the new twenty, but let's be honest—your skin might be saying and feeling otherwise! Your epidermis may not be as supple as it once was and new problems might be arising when it comes to its texture and appearance. To tackle the decrease in your skin's elasticity, firmness, and moisture, choose products specifically based on your skin type (see Chapter 2). Also, add an antioxidant-rich serum to help stimulate the growth of new cells.

As for skin issues, you may start to notice a case of keratosis, a skin condition that is characterized by a rough, bumpy texture on your arms, chest, back, or even your hairline. Exfoliation and using products that include alpha hydroxy acid (AHA) and beta hydroxy acid (BHA) are very helpful at keeping keratosis at bay.

You may also notice couperose skin, which is redness and distended capillaries caused by weakening of the capillary walls. Stress and pollution are major triggers. To ease the discoloration, try some of the at-home tricks in Chapter 5 to decrease this complaint.

And last, those dreaded wrinkles, lines, furrows, and nasal labial folds (parentheses lines around the mouth) may start developing. They are caused by a buildup of free radicals (external pollution and cells exacerbating) that will create indentations in the skin. To help "plump" up these problem areas, try using a cream with hyaluronic acid or use GABA or myrtle leaf in extract form. In addition to using antiaging, ingredient-specific products, you can find some additional helpful solutions in Chapter 2.

In Your Fifties

Welcome to the half-century mark! Of course, with age comes wisdom . . . and unfortunately skin that is starting to show signs of wear and tear. So it's time to do all you can to improve the texture and tone of your advanced skin. This means using exceptional antiaging products daily to look your best.

Of course, one of the biggest signs of aging is a loss of elasticity in your epidermis in the form of sagging, loose, or crepey skin caused from skin movement damage, sun, or skin irritation. To fix this dilemma, try adding more cardio to your routine to build muscles and tighten up your epidermis as well as adding some of the antiaging foods from Chapter 4 into your diet. You'll be amazed what a little gelatin can do; the more often you can include it in your diet, the better.

You may also notice more hyperpigmentation, or brown discoloration, from melanin production due to sun irritation or overuse of doctor-prescribed medications. See Chapters 2 and 7 (lemons can do wonders!) for ways to help lighten the spots.

One last problem to look out for is hyperkeratinization, which is the massive buildup of dead cells in a concentrated area of your skin. Gentle exfoliation twice a day, along with deep moisturization, will lead to a slowing of this ongoing effect.

In Your Sixties and Beyond

Just when you think you've seen it all, along comes a new set of skin issues that seem to appear just as you enter your swinging sixties. At this stage of the game, you've probably encountered a plethora of skin problems over the course of your life and now have to deal with the consequences of issues that have been building up for decades that may or may not have surfaced. But the good news is that there's absolutely a solution to any new challenge that crops up.

You may start to notice more rosacea on your face, which is chronic redness, small papules, and pustules that will need to be managed, exfoliated, and extracted to avoid enlarged pores or elasticity challenges. Adding certain foods to your diet (see Chapter 4) and trying a few of my at-home masks (see Chapter 5) may help.

Asphyxiated skin could also be a problem. Smokers primarily have this condition from a lack of oxygen, characterized by clogged pores and wrinkles, as well as skin that is dull and lifeless looking. See Chapter 5 for some brightening tips!

And last, medical conditions, such as heart conditions, epilepsy, diabetes, contact dermatitis, lupus, and other medication situations can exacerbate aging skin. Fortifying your skin internally and externally with the same actives will help stabilize your skin, so coordinating the right combination is key.

8

Into the Real World

YOU KNOW HOW TO ORGANIZE your life and find ways to retrofit your environment, how to calibrate your stress levels, how to consume and cook food, and how to spot the right ingredients in the products you use to benefit your skin and body the most. And now, to round out your journey, I want to put all of those elements into play by showing you how to utilize them in some of the most personal occasions of your life. Looking good and feeling good are synonymous, so take what you've learned so far and read on to see how it all comes together in any major life moment or situation you may encounter.

Getting Red-Carpet Ready—
for Any Occasion!

Hollywood is full of red-carpet events with celebrities who look picture-perfect. It takes a bit of work, but the end result leaves them all glowing and beautiful. You may not have a premiere or a gala to attend, but I'm sure there are plenty of dressy occasions you have coming up in your own life (weddings, bar mitzvahs, or formal parties) where you want to go the extra mile to rival any celebrity on a press line.

So here is the VIP beauty plan I give my celebrity clients to ensure their skin is spectacularly eye-catching on their big night. It's a plan you can easily use to prepare yourself to look red-carpet ready for any event in your life.

Day 1

This program starts seven days before your event. The first day is the most important, because you're going to jump-start your entire system to get yourself moving in the right direction. You'll be detoxifying your body and changing your behavior to begin your skintervention right from the starting block! By following this plan, within a week your skin should feel more hydrated and taut—but you have to stick to the program.

Day 1 is a minicleanse in which you should consume no more than 1,000 calories. On this first day you'll also want to exfoliate twice—once in the morning and once at night. If you have sensitive skin, exfoliate just once. A deep exfoliation with a proven product is necessary, because it will slough off buildup and excess oils, and trigger your skin to start creating new cells.

You should also drink at least 64 ounces of water, which will help to flush toxins from your body and supply moisture to your cells. You should eat a total of one tablespoon of extra-virgin olive oil, as well as foods high in vitamins A, C, and E, which are high in antioxidants. And remember to limit your salt intake! The less sodium in your food, the less bloated you'll be.

The menus below are samples only, so feel free to mix and match foods according to your tastes and lifestyle. Most of the menus range from 1,200 to 1,400 calories, but you can adjust them based on your current weight and health needs.

Breakfast
✓ Egg-white omelet made with 4 egg whites, 1/2 cup fresh spinach leaves, 2 teaspoons minced onion, 2 diced mushrooms, and 1 teaspoon olive oil to coat pan.
✓ 1 orange
✓ unsweetened green tea

Lunch
✓ Salad made from 1 cup Romaine lettuce, 1/2 tomato, 1/4 onion, and 1/4 cucumber, dressed with 1 teaspoon of olive oil and 2 teaspoons balsamic vinegar. Top salad with 3 ounces of grilled chicken, fish, or light tofu.

Afternoon Snack
✓ 1 cup low-fat yogurt with 6 unsalted almonds or walnuts

Dinner

✓ 4 ounces of grilled or baked salmon with store-bought or homemade salsa (To make the salsa, dice 1/4 cucumber, 1/4 tomato, 1/4 onion, and 1/4 mango or peach; mix with the juice of 1/2 lime or 1/2 lemon. Add red pepper flakes, chili powder, ginger, and/or garlic to taste.)

✓ 1 cup broccoli or spinach (sauté with 1 teaspoon olive oil, chopped garlic or garlic powder, a splash of lemon, and pepper)

Day 2

Day 2 is a day for repair. You need to eat 60 grams of protein today to give your body the essential amino acids it needs to repair skin cells (eggs, skinless chicken breast, tofu, and almonds are good choices). You should have another 60–64 ounces of water, as well as a tablespoon of extra-virgin olive oil. Repeat the same skin routine as Day 1 (exfoliate twice a day; once a day for those with sensitive skin). From this point on, avoid saturated fats and greasy, fried foods.

Breakfast

✓ Omelet made with 4 eggs and 1/2 cup spinach or red pepper (use 1 teaspoon of olive oil to coat the pan or spray with Pam)

✓ 1 orange or 1/2 cup strawberries

✓ 1 cup green tea unsweetened

Morning Snack

✓ 1 piece Mini Babybel Light Original Cheese

✓ 1 small apple or pear

Lunch

✓ 4 ounces of lean deli turkey or skinless chicken breast in 1/2 whole wheat pita pocket; stuff sandwich with spinach leaves, shredded carrots, and sliced tomato; dress with mustard.

✓ 1 hard-boiled egg

✓ 1/2 cup sliced strawberries or 1 small orange

Snack

✓ 1 6-ounce container Chobani Greek yogurt with 10 almonds

Dinner

✓ 4 ounces lean sirloin steak, grilled

✓ 1 portobello mushroom cap brushed with olive oil, sea salt, and pepper, grilled

✓ 1 side salad with 1 teaspoon of olive oil and lemon or balsamic vinegar; add 1 tablespoon of chopped walnuts or almonds

Day 3

Day 3 will follow the same skin and water routine as Day 2 (drink between 60–64 ounces of water and exfoliate once for sensitive skin; twice for all other skin types). Consume no more than 1,000 calories today; have one tablespoon of extra-virgin olive oil; eat foods high in vitamins A, C, and E.

Breakfast

✓ Egg-white omelet made with 1 egg and 2 egg whites with 1/2 cup green or red pepper (use 1 teaspoon of olive oil to coat the pan or spray it with Pam)

✓ 1 orange

✓ unsweetened green tea

Morning Snack

✓ 1 piece Mini Babybel Light Original Cheese

✓ 1 small apple

Lunch

✓ Large salad made with 1 cup of greens with 1/2 tomato,
   1/2 cucumber, and 1/2 red pepper (dress with 1 teaspoon
   of balsamic vinegar mixed with 1 teaspoon of olive oil)

✓ 4 ounces of grilled chicken, fish, or light tofu

✓ 1 small apple or 1/2 cup watermelon

✓ Water or unsweetened green tea

Afternoon Snack

✓ 1 6-ounce container low-fat yogurt

Dinner

✓ 1 cup steamed broccoli

✓ 1 tablespoon light butter with canola oil (such as Land O'Lakes)

✓ 4 ounces grilled or baked tilapia or grouper with lemon or salsa

✓ Water or unsweetened green tea

Day 4

Today you want to spot treat all your problem areas, including blemishes, sun spots, and deep wrinkles. Blemishes can be targeted by a trip to the esthetician, but sun spots are slightly trickier and can be managed by products with high amounts of kojic acid (anything over 4 percent). Continue drinking 60–64 ounces of water each day and eat one tablespoon of extra-virgin olive oil. Your diet should be high in omega-3s (like salmon) to help power-pack your body with antioxidants.

Breakfast

- ✓ 1 piece of multigrain or high-fiber toast
- ✓ 1 tablespoon of jam or jelly
- ✓ 1/2 cup of strawberries
- ✓ Water or unsweetened green tea

Morning Snack

- ✓ 1 tablespoon of peanut butter
- ✓ 1 small apple

Lunch

- ✓ Salad with 1 cup of shredded romaine, 1/2 cup of chopped green or red pepper, 1 celery stalk, chopped, 1/2 tomato, sliced; dress with 1 teaspoon of balsamic vinegar and 1 teaspoon of olive oil
- ✓ 4 ounces of canned tuna packed in water

Afternoon Snack

- ✓ 1/2 cup of sliced strawberries
- ✓ 6 ounces fat-free or low-fat yogurt

Dinner

- ✓ 4 ounces High-energy Salmon Steak (see recipe on page 83)
- ✓ 1 small baked potato, plain (dress with a few teaspoons of salsa or one teaspoon of sour cream)
- ✓ 1 cup steamed or sautéed asparagus or spinach with 1 teaspoon olive oil and spritz of lemon
- ✓ 1 small side salad with balsamic vinegar and 1 teaspoon olive oil; add 1 tablespoon chopped almonds, walnuts, or pecans

Day 5

Continue using the spot treatment method from Day 4, drink 60–64 ounces of water, and consume 1 tablespoon of extra-virgin olive oil as well as foods high in vitamins A, C, and E.

Breakfast
- ✓ 1 cup General Mills Chex Multi-bran cereal
- ✓ 4 ounces skim milk
- ✓ 4 ounces orange juice or 1 small orange

Morning Snack
- ✓ 1/2 cup grapes
- ✓ 1 piece of Mini Babybel Light cheese

Lunch
- ✓ 4 ounces of skinless chicken breast in a multigrain wrap; layer with spinach leaves, shredded carrots, and dress with mustard or olive oil and balsamic dressing
- ✓ 1/2 cup of strawberries or carrot sticks

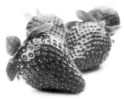

Afternoon Snack
- ✓ 6 ounces nonfat yogurt or one 8-ounce carton of enriched Vanilla Soy Milk

Dinner
- ✓ 4 ounces lean sirloin steak, grilled
- ✓ 1 cup of cooked wild rice
- ✓ Side salad with 1 teaspoon olive oil and balsamic vinegar

Day 6

Give yourself a light exfoliation in the morning. Continue using the spot treatment method from Day 4, drink 60–64 ounces of water, and have 1 tablespoon extra-virgin olive oil, as well as foods high in vitamins A, C, and E.

Breakfast

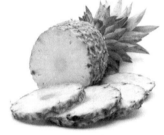

- ✓ 1/2 cup pineapple
- ✓ 1/2 cup fat-free yogurt
- ✓ 1 scrambled egg on 1 slice high-fiber toast

Lunch

- ✓ 1 whole wheat pita with 3 ounces of skinless chicken breast
- ✓ Side salad with 1 cup lettuce, 1/2 tomato, 1/2 cucumber, and 1/4 onion with 1 teaspoon olive oil and balsamic vinegar
- ✓ 1 small apple

Afternoon Snack

- ✓ 6 ounces fat-free or low-fat yogurt
- ✓ 1/2 cup strawberries

Dinner

- ✓ Chicken tortilla made with 4 ounces skinless chicken breast, 1 tablespoon hot sauce, 2 tablespoons canned kidney beans, 1 small red bell pepper, chopped, and 1/2 onion, chopped, on a soft multigrain tortilla
- ✓ Side salad made with 2 cups of greens and veggies; dress with 1 teaspoon of olive oil and 2 teaspoons of balsamic vinegar.

Day 7

Continue using the spot treatment method from Day 4, drink 60–64 ounces of water, and have 1 tablespoon extra-virgin olive oil and foods high in vitamins A, C, and E. One hour prior to putting on your dress, stop drinking water to reduce bloating.

Breakfast
- ✓ 1 piece of multigrain or high-fiber toast
- ✓ 1 tablespoon of jam or jelly
- ✓ 1/2 cup of strawberries
- ✓ unsweetened green tea

Morning Snack
- ✓ 1 tablespoon of peanut butter
- ✓ 1 small apple

Lunch
- ✓ Salad with 1 cup of shredded romaine, 1/2 cup of chopped green or red pepper, 1 celery stalk, chopped, 1/2 tomato, sliced; dress with 1 teaspoon of balsamic vinegar and 1 teaspoon of olive oil
- ✓ 4 ounces of canned tuna packed in water

Afternoon Snack
- ✓ 1/2 cup of sliced strawberries or blueberries
- ✓ 6 ounces fat-free or low-fat yogurt

Dinner
- ✓ 4 ounces of grilled or baked salmon with lemon
- ✓ 1 cup steamed or sautéed asparagus or spinach with 1 teaspoon olive oil and spritz of lemon
- ✓ 1 small side salad with balsamic vinegar and 1 teaspoon olive oil; add 1 tablespoon low-fat feta cheese or walnuts

By the end of the week, your skin should be looking flawless and red-carpet ready!

Close Encounters

Over the years, the number one insight I've gotten from women is that no woman thinks her skin is good enough and says there is always room for improvement. I haven't really met one who says, "I have genetically beautiful skin and I never have to do a thing to it." They always think that even if they're told they have perfect skin, even some of the most beautiful actresses in Hollywood, they will tell me there is a flaw of some sort. So you're not alone if being in any type of situation where you're going to be sitting in close proximity to someone brings on a serious case of nerves and concerns about your appearance.

These situations can range from having a dinner in a restaurant to sitting in a meeting with your boss, or even going in for a job interview with a stranger. Being in any type of environment and having a close-space conversation is the number one most conscious moment that a lot of women have and is what they feel the most insecure about. Fortunately, there are ways to help make these situations less nerve-racking and more comfortable, allowing you to shine and put your best foot forward.

In addition to doing things to help yourself internally, if you haven't completely fixed your skin challenge, there are ways to mask it so that you'll feel more confident during that close-up conversation. My first suggestion is to choose an environment for the meeting where the areas of your skin that trouble you are not on display. If you feel like your oily skin will be acting up or you'd rather not have someone notice the makeup you're using to cover up your acne scars, try to pick a situation where the lighting is going to be more flattering, such as a place with dim or low lighting, which can be found in most restaurants. That way, the focus won't necessarily be a bright light shining on your skin and will land on your winning smile instead.

The same goes for people with genetically large pores. Before your important meeting, try some of my tips in Chapter 5 to help close them up, like using products containing lactic acid or vitamins A and C, or even dousing your face with ice-cold water before you go out. Then make sure you meet in a place with adjusted lighting to deflect the focus off your pores. In addition, during your meeting, try to project confidence in your voice and not worry about your skin challenges. If you're not worried about them, the people you're with probably won't perceive that you have them either!

As a rule, don't ever talk about the challenges you currently have on your skin because that is what people pick up on, and that's when they'll actually start to focus on them. During your close-up conversation, try to avoid saying things like, "Oh, I look so gross" or even "Oh my gosh, my mascara is running." Don't ever say anything negative, because that's all the person you're with is going to see and focus on. Draw their attention elsewhere and showcase things you feel confident about.

First-Date Jitters

On first dates, not only are you wondering what to wear, whether you should go someplace casual or not, or if the person is going to like you, but you want to make sure that if you're going to get up close and personal with someone new, your skin woes aren't going to be a hindrance to you completely being yourself. That's why it's important to look and feel your best so you'll make that always-memorable first impression.

For a first date that you have a week or so to plan for, try some of the things I suggest for a bride approaching her wedding day (more details below). Do some gentle exfoliation and maybe even squeeze in a light facial. Drink lots of water to keep your skin clear, and if you're worried about bloating, try cutting out salt and carbs a few days before your big date.

If you only have a few days to prepare for a first date, make sure you do your exfoliation properly and create that look of flawless canvassing so your skin can correctly absorb products after your pores are closed (see Chapters 3, 5, and 7 for suggestions). And if you're up for it, you can try to do a twenty-four-hour cleanse to have your skin looking its best and to get that naturally contoured look on your face.

But if you're really nervous, no matter what skin condition you have, try not to worry, and concentrate on doing things that boost your confidence. Remind yourself of the features and assets you really like about yourself and focus on those. Skin conditions will come and go, but the core of who you are will always remain the same. So shake off those nerves and shine from the inside out. Your date won't be able to resist your glowing charm!

And the Prom Queen Is . . .

The prom is one of the most anticipated events in high school, and every girl hopes the night will be perfect . . . and of course this includes looking absolutely amazing. As a result, many girls typically start worrying about how they'll look months in advance. It's almost like a wedding in a way! Sound about right?

Even before you have a prom date, you're probably thinking about the perfect dress. And most likely, it'll be one that shows off your arms, neck, face, and even parts of your back. Of course, you want to have perfect skin that night, but as with many teenage girls, acne breakouts are quite common. Fortunately, if you start early enough, you can have clear skin by the big night.

If your skin tends to break out a lot, start by incorporating clarifying foods into your diet a few months in advance. These will be foods that contain a high level of vitamin A, as well as polyphenols like pomegranate and goji berries (see Chapter 4). If you are trying this a few months before the prom and can't holistically break your acne cycle within two weeks and aren't seeing a clarifying benefit, make an appointment to see an esthetician or a dermatologist who can prescribe a topical medication.

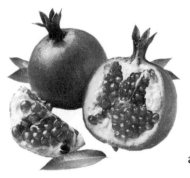

By doing this early enough, you can figure out if your skin-care routine might make you dry, flaky, or irritated before the big night arrives. Experimenting with your diet and routine two or three months before will get you on the right regimen so your prom night is everything you always envisioned.

Wiping Out Wedding Day Skin Woes

It is a necessity that you start paying attention to your skin care one month before your wedding day (or two months if you have challenged skin, such as blemishes or redness). It is as important as finalizing the seating arrangements or the flowers. It's just something else you should add to your list of things to do before the big day arrives. It might sound crazy, but remember that the number one thing people are going to see and remember from your wedding is how you looked and the happy glow you radiated all night long. The wedding is going to be over, the flowers are going to wither away, and the cake is going to be eaten, but your wedding pictures are going to live forever. And who wouldn't want to look and feel their absolute best on one of the most memorable days of their life?

Four weeks before your wedding you should get all of your major treatments done: your major dermabrasion if you need it; your extractions, peels, and waxing—all of the things that could possibly cause skin challenges. You don't want to get these procedures done too close to your wedding day, just in case your skin has a bad reaction. However, if you have these treatments done and they don't cause serious redness, skin damage, hives, or anything like that, then you can still do them up to two weeks before your wedding. These treatments will create new and undamaged skin, so when you apply your makeup on your wedding day, the application will go on flawlessly, and you'll look amazing in your pictures.

Three weeks before your nuptials you should figure out what you want your makeup to look like on your wedding day. Try to determine what the weather is going to be like: humid or dry or a chance of rain, and choose makeup and products that will work best on your skin in those conditions. You want things that won't fade as the night goes on and, of course, be sure the mascara you choose is not going to run from all of your happy tears! You want makeup that you're not going to have to touch up a lot throughout the night after it's done the first time. The more touch-ups you have, the more you'll ruin the contouring and everything else that the makeup artist (or you) spent so much time creating.

This is the time where you should be serious about drinking cleansing water—and more water in general—to help you detoxify and give you the radiant skin you desire. During this time, a healthy diet and proper hydration will cause a beneficial, synergistic effect which will continue all the way up until your wedding day.

You'll also want to use products that are going to clarify your skin (see Chapter 2 for skin type specifics). Over the next few weeks, don't worry about age-defying products. Don't worry about replenishing products. Your goal is clear, porcelain skin on your entire body, because like most women, on your wedding day you'll most likely have your face, décolleté, arms, and back totally showing. Therefore, you'll want everything on your body to be cleansed.

Two weeks before you tie the knot, you should run through a

few hair and makeup trials to get them down pat so that they will be perfect on your big day. In addition, it's important that your makeup artist and your skin-care specialist work together to find the right system for your skin. Surprisingly, this is the number one thing most women do *not* do two weeks before their wedding date, outside of eating and drinking right and exercising. If you are your own esthetician, you need to tell your makeup artist what products you are using so your makeup artist knows how those products will interact with the products he or she is going to use on you that day. You want to make sure all of the products will work in harmony. The reason for this is because a lot of shadows and powders won't absorb fully or stay completely on skin that is too saturated with products, and some foundations won't work on top of certain skin-care creams and lotions. Most spray foundations will work on top of treated skin, but they can peel and flake very easily if not used with the right combination of skin-care products.

You also want to properly bronze with a skin-care highlighter, which is any product containing light-reflectors such as mica, pearl, or flonac, rather than using a color foundation bronzing product. The reason I say this is because the number one thing women hate in their wedding photos is the look of overcontoured skin, and that's what most makeup artists do because they think brides want that look for their wedding. But the artist can achieve the same contoured effect by using highly reflective skin-care sticks and/or creams on top of makeup versus using an actual contour cosmetic.

Also, this is the week you should get your hair cut—not the week before your wedding. Most women will get their hair colored and cut the week of their wedding because they want fresh color. But if something happens that week and some of the color accidentally drips onto your face, it will stain the new skin you've been working so hard to create, and you will end up seeing it in your wedding pictures, especially around your hairline.

One week before your wedding you should get a very light facial and do a gentle exfoliation, rather than a heavy exfoliation, twice a day. You should also consistently exfoliate every area of your skin that is going to show when you wear your bridal gown.

Three days prior to your wedding, you should drink lots of water, of course, but also eat a lot of fish and vegetables. Also, I don't like to be the Carb Police but do not eat any carbs—not only for your waistline, but also for the translucent glow it will give your skin. I know it's difficult to cut out all the carbs, but it will be so worth it. You can have a little bit of sugar, but if you want glowing skin, cut out those carbs!

And overall, try to get lots of sound, restful sleep. A good eight or nine hours a night is what your body and skin need to recharge. Exercise regularly, try to avoid excess exposure to extremes of temperature, limit your intake of caffeine and alcohol, and if possible, try to keep your stress level to a minimum. I know it's not an easy task, but your skin will be thanking you later!

One last thing—*do not* go tanning! Strapless wedding gowns and backless bridesmaids' dresses are driving brides to insist on taking rounds on tanning beds as part of wedding preparation.

But friends shouldn't make friends tan! Skin cancer caused by tanning is dangerously on the rise. Brides who think they need a "base" tan to look stunning at their wedding should think twice before going into a tanning booth. Tanning only leads to problems in the future, such as skin cancer and wrinkles. And, of course, a cosmetic cream or powdered bronzer is a great and healthier alternative!

And remember—the harmful effects of tanning last far longer than posing for wedding photos. Young people tanning today probably won't see immediate skin damage and falsely think there's no problem. Yet risk for skin cancer accumulates over time. So let your natural skin shine, and that way, when you walk down the aisle, guests will focus on your glowing, healthy skin and radiant smile and not how tan you are.

Reunions: I Haven't Seen You in Ages!

If you are going to your high school or college reunion, summer camp reunion, or family reunion, the one thing that's probably at the top of your concern list is how everyone is going to think you look. And of course you want to look as good as—if not better than—you did the last time you saw everyone, right?

The first step in doing that is examining your pictures of when you saw these people last. It doesn't matter how long ago it was; just take out the pictures and see how you looked and ask yourself if you liked how you appeared back then. Did you like your skin? Did you like your physique? Did you like your hair? What did you want to change at that time, and what do you want to change now, if anything at all? Make a list and then go back into this book and augment those things within the chapters to create an end result that you're happy with. That way, when you walk into that reunion and do your reveal, you'll have the self-assurance to chat with anyone and be as confident as you can be.

You want to get that compliment of "You haven't aged a day!" or "You look even better now than you did then!" Maybe someone will say, "You look even better with age." And the best chance you have of hearing any of these things is by looking at your past photos and seeing if you are actually trending that way and if you aren't, actually doing something about it by using this book as a tool to get there.

And much like my advice to a bride, skip the tanning booths before the reunion. Having a fake glow isn't worth the risk of damaging your skin for a lifetime.

Conclusion

· ·

BY NOW YOU SHOULD BE ARMED with all the information and strategies you need to be the best and healthiest version of yourself. You can live your best life and be confidently gorgeous from the inside out! And as you can see, by changing even the smallest part of your daily routine, you'll experience a noticeable difference in the way you see yourself and how others see you.

As you can see, my suggestions, hints, and advice can be applied to anyone—from a high school student in a small town to a vibrant grandmother who loves to travel, and even Hollywood actors and actresses who have some of the most beautiful faces in film and television! It is all information that's easy to digest (sometimes literally!) and even easier to apply.

Actress Mila Kunis noticed an instant difference in her appearance by making just a few small changes to her skin-care routine after our first appointment. And if I can do that for a woman who is in the spotlight as much as she is, then I know I can do it for each of you. Mila recently said something that is exactly on point with the message I'm trying to get across, and I'd like to share it with you.

I believe healthier and clearer skin gives a person more confidence, and that's what Scott-Vincent Borba and his inside-out philosophy are all about. I was very inspired by the tips and tricks he taught me to help keep my skin looking its best, and I can honestly say that they work! For example, I tried exfoliating my face first before I cleansed it, and right away I noticed that my skin felt cleaner, and I could immediately see the difference! Even doing the little things that Scott-Vincent suggests can make a huge improvement.

When things in this book work for you, you'll be happier, and when you're happy, that's all you need. It's the light at the end of the tunnel. If you try things and they don't work, that's okay— other things will. It's not going to hurt you to try different tactics, and at the end of the day, you'll be healthier. So if you know it works, you know there are going to be good results, and you know it's all healthy and there's nothing bad for you about it, why not give it a try? I certainly did, and my skin is thanking me for it!

Before you read on, take a moment to reflect back on how far you've come. Pull out your before photo and then look at yourself in the mirror. Do you see an improvement? Did you alter those things you set out to change? Hopefully the answer is "yes"! And now you know what to do holistically and internally to keep the external parts of you looking the way you want—and the pitfalls to avoid so you can stay looking that way.

Looking Good for Yourself

At the end of the day, you probably want to look good for yourself, not just for those around you. If you feel good about yourself and you think you look good and you have inner confidence, that's going to make dealing with all of the other obstacles you encounter in your life, or things you want to fix within yourself, a bit easier. Everything in your life starts with you—what you want for yourself, how you feel, and, ultimately, how you perceive yourself in the outside world. And I'm telling you, if you really make the effort to alter those things that are holding you back from feeling your best, you'll notice a big difference in how that overall picture will change for the better.

Start by staring into the mirror and deciding if a physical change will make you feel happier. If so, narrow down what it is and then say, "I love myself for what I am, but I want to change this particular thing about myself, and that's what I want to focus on." Then go back into this book and highlight those areas that are most important to you and focus on those things—screw all the other stuff! That's what I tell all of my clients, even the biggest celebrities in Hollywood. If you don't care that you get a blemish once in a while, or that you have acne on your hairline from perimenopause, or that you have dry patches when you are PMSing, then just focus on the issue you care about the most and let all that other stuff just run its course.

Wear clothes that highlight your best assets. Choose colors that give you confidence. Find the right combination of makeup that makes you look in the mirror and smile at who you see staring back at you. And no matter who is going to see you that day, knowing you feel great about how you look will give you the self-assurance you need to accomplish anything you set out to do. Positivity breeds positivity, so don't let anything hold you back!

By tackling things one at a time, you'll find that bit by bit, you'll become happier with how you look, and as a result, you'll be happier with who you are overall. People in your life may be telling you to change things because they don't like them, but ultimately, and more important, you should want to change things on your body for yourself to make you feel the best you can possibly be.

And Finally . . .

As you embark on this journey in search of the right internal and external process that's going to give you the skin you've been looking for, you really need to challenge yourself. You have to take that before-and-after picture. Pay attention to your body. Listen to what it's saying and what it needs. Get other people involved so they can support and help you as you go through this challenge.

Start simple and figure out the first (and easiest) thing that you can do that will affect the current challenges you have; then decide what the second thing will be; and so on. Take these steps one at a time and don't overwhelm yourself with multiple changes at once. Decide what you can make happen and just do it. Then let someone know that you hit that first finish line and that's what's going to get you to the next step. Having a support team is key! The more you do, the more you project out there what you want; and the more people you have involved with you in this process, the more change you are going to see in yourself, internally as well as externally.

My mother Evelyn and my sisters Sandy and Stacy are three of the most beautiful women that I have ever met. They have embraced my philosophies and not only look and feel younger but are evangelists because my methods actually work. Even if you don't do every single tactic, doing just one will make such a difference that you will be yearning to tackle other tips, which will help build on the good you've already achieved!

So here are my final bits of advice: Go through this book and mark the important pages with a sticky tab as a reminder of how and when to do things. Next, I suggest going through the steps to make the changes you want, and when you see the results, write down how it makes you feel (maybe in a journal), so you'll always remember that positive feeling and experience. That way, if in the worst case you fall off course and that problem resurfaces, being able to go back and reread that feeling of elation from your success will recharge you to get back to regaining the changes you loved and embodied.

Also, if you are more private and don't want to enlist people to engage in the challenge with you, then my suggestion is that when you succeed in each phase of my book, reward yourself with something you love—a new outfit, seeing a movie, going to a concert—whatever is going to make you happy from the inside out. And I mean it. Do it. It's time to make YOU the priority and not everyone else around you. I'm giving you the permission to make yourself the focus, so the changes you make within yourself can be felt positively by all the people around you!

And people *will* notice—I promise. The true proof of change is when you see the waiter lingering at your table for an extra minute, a stranger looking you right in the eyes and smiling, or even your partner noticing something more detailed about you that you wouldn't normally hear as a compliment. That is your inner and outer beauty being admired. That is what made me feel so wonderful when I went through my personal change and a random, loving compliment was paid to me. I still treasure that, and you will too.

"No" is no longer in your vocabulary, and anyone who doubts you must be used as fodder to make you work harder! Use any negative energy that comes your way to your benefit, and make your transformation even quicker and more positive!

And always remember, I am your biggest fan, and that is why I wrote this book. I believe in you, and if I can make such a dramatic change with *my* life, then *anyone* can do it. Prove to yourself that the beauty of your soul will be revealed outwardly when you successfully complete your amazing and life-changing skintervention!

Index

About the Author

Popular with consumers, audiences, and media alike, BORBA founder and CEO Scott-Vincent Borba has earned a solid reputation as a prescient thinker and beauty business visionary. In developing first-of-their-kind beauty products for his company and treating the skin from both the inside and out, he is indeed changing the way people think about skin care.

It begins with Scott-Vincent's philosophy of building beauty from the inside out. For him, health and beauty are one and the same. To encourage healthy skin from within, there are BORBA Nutraceuticals. For the outside, the company offers a full range of BORBA Cosmeceuticals that deliver potent problem-solving, antioxidant-rich formulas topically.

Since launching BORBA in 2004, Scott-Vincent has nimbly steered BORBA from one success to another. Since his first appearance on QVC in 2006, for example, Scott-Vincent has performed numerous hour-long BORBA shows in front of millions of viewers—often selling out his products.

The youngest of five children, Scott-Vincent is originally from a small farming town in California. "I received unequivocal guidance and support from my parents," he remembers. "They encouraged my ambitions to escape the constraints of the small town and create something bigger, something significant of my life."

During college, Scott-Vincent worked as a Ford model and participated in major fashion campaigns and runway shows, including Calvin Klein and Versace. He earned his B.S. degree from Santa Clara University and is a licensed esthetician. His subsequent move to Los Angeles was an education in itself in the art and science of the beauty business. There he built career successes in both prestige and mass-market sectors in product development, branding, and marketing for companies such as Hard Candy, Neutrogena, P&G/Wella/Sebastian, Shiseido/Joico, and Murad before setting out on his own as founder of BORBA and cofounder of e.l.f. (eyes, lips, face) Cosmetics.

But the biggest turning point for Scott-Vincent came when his father took ill and he went on a loving quest to find a more holistic way to help him improve his health. During his research, Scott-Vincent discovered the founding principle of his inside/out philosophy, which in turn became the catalyst for the next phase of his personal and professional life.

In addition, Scott-Vincent is an active supporter of and the global spokesperson for Covenant House California, a nonprofit organization providing food, shelter, life-skills counseling, and education for youth in need.

"What I particularly love about beauty," concludes Scott-Vincent Borba, "is that it sits right in the middle between science and fashion, drawing inspiration and content from both. You get the rigor and structure of one combined with the glamour and promise of the other. For me, that's the most intriguing and exciting thing in the world."

Please visit www.scottvincentborba.com or www.facebook.com/SVB to learn more about Scott-Vincent Borba and BORBA products.